VASCULITIS IN PRACTICE - AN UPDATE ON SPECIAL SITUATIONS-CLINICAL AND THERAPEUTIC CONSIDERATIONS

Edited by **Reem Hamdy Abdellatif Mohammed**

Vasculitis In Practice-An Update on Special Situations-Clinical and Therapeutic Considerations
http://dx.doi.org/10.5772/intechopen.69793
Edited by Reem Hamdy Abdellatif Mohammed

Contributors

Sophia Lionaki, John Boletis, Daniel Cacione, Munekazu Yamakuchi, Sushil Panta, Teruto Hashiguchi, Reem Hamdy A Mohammed

Notice

First published in London, United Kingdom, 2018 by IntechOpen
IntechOpen is the global imprint of INTECHOPEN LIMITED, registered in England and Wales, registration number: 11086078, The Shard, 25th floor, 32 London Bridge Street
London, SE19SG – United Kingdom
Printed in Croatia

British Library Cataloguing-in-Publication Data
A catalogue record for this book is available from the British Library

Additional hard copies can be obtained from orders@intechopen.com

Vasculitis In Practice-An Update on Special Situations-Clinical and Therapeutic Considerations, Edited by Reem Hamdy Abdellatif Mohammed

p. cm.

Print ISBN 978-1-78923-698-9
Online ISBN 978-1-78923-699-6

For EU product safety concerns:
IN TECH d.o.o., Prolaz Marije Krucifikse Kozulić 3, 51000 Rijeka, Croatia,
info@intechopen.com or visit our website at intechopen.com.

Meet the editor

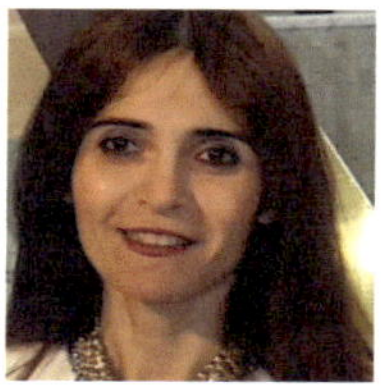

Dr. Reem Hamdy Abdellatif Mohammed is a professor of Rheumatology, Clinical Immunology and Rehabilitation at the Kasr Alainy School of Medicine, Cairo University Hospitals, Cairo University, Egypt. Prof Dr. Reem Hamdy graduated with her MB, BSCh, MSc, MD in rheumatology, clinical immunology, rehabilitation, and PhD in rheumatology and immunology from the Department of Rheumatology and Rehabilitation, Kasr Alainy School of Medicine, Cairo University. She is also a Fellow of the Royal College of Physicians (FRCP), UK.
Dr. Reem has been serving as an editor and recognized international reviewer of a number of reputable international medical journals and is a co-author for a number of book publications and international speaker in the field of rheumatology and immunology.

Contents

Preface

The term "vasculitis" describes an inflammatory process that involves the blood vessels and contributes to vascular damage. Autoimmunity, infections, drugs, and malignancies have been considered among potential etio-pathogenic factors. In vasculitis, the inflammation might develop in either a systemic or organ-specific form and might exist as an independent pathology usually defined as "primary vasculitis" or as a presentation of an existing primary pathology, that is, "secondary vasculitis".

Owing to the heterogeneous patterns of vascular involvement, most importantly the vessel size, the organ/organs affected, and the nature of the inflammatory process, the clinical classification of vasculitis is a major challenge. In 1994, the Chapel Hill Consensus Conference designed a classification based on the vessel size; however, the proposed classification wasn't enough to provide sufficient differential diagnostic outlines in real-life practice.

In 2012, the Chapel Hill Consensus Conference revised the 1994 classification towards a more precise sorting of vasculitis that is relevant to clinical practice. In their classification, the panel provided a more practical approach considering different aetiologies that might contribute to the pathology, the nature of the pathology, and the vessel size. Interestingly, the classification introduced new terms based on clinical evidence and these terms included variable vessel vasculitis, single organ vasculitis, and vasculitis due to possible aetiologies.

The identification, classification, and management of vasculitis in specific clinical situations are the focus of this book, including an update on proposed therapeutic strategies in an evidence-based approach.

Acknowledgment

To my beloved, supporting family—my husband Hesham, my daughter Maya and my son Kareem—thank you for everything you have done to make this possible. I wish to make you proud of me forever.

Professor Reem Hamdy Abdellatif Mohammed
Professor of Rheumatology and Clinical immunology
Department of Rheumatology and Rehabilitation
Kasr Alainy School of Medicine
Cairo University, Cairo, Egypt

Section 1

Introduction

Chapter 1

Introductory Chapter: Vasculitis

Reem Hamdy A. Mohammed

Additional information is available at the end of the chapter

http://dx.doi.org/10.5772/intechopen.79560

1. Introduction

The nomenclature "Vasculitis" is a pathologic term that refers to an inflammatory process affecting a vessel wall, the inflammation leads to fibrinoid necrosis and vessel wall damage. The inflammatory process takes place in either isolate or mixed forms synchronously or sequentially with interruption of the blood flow to vital tissues giving protean presentations. It is the territorial and developmental characteristics of the vessels that determine the patterns and the after comings of the pathology. The etiology of the disease remains largely unexplored. On the one hand, when vessel inflammation exists as an independent pathology, it is usually classified as primary vasculitis; on the other hand, if vessel inflammation develops as a part of an existing primary pathology, it is classified as secondary vasculitis. An evidence-based approach to the classification of vasculitis has been challenged by the uniquely heterogeneous pattern of the inflammatory process, the confusing serology, non-uniform response to therapy, and poorly identified prognostic markers [1].

In 1994, the Chapel Hill Consensus Conference designed a nomenclature classification of vasculitis based on the size of the affected vessel [2, 3]. Clinical and research evidences have proven that considering vessel caliber as the sole determining factor for a multiplicity of heterogeneous consequences seems a rather simple hypothesis for a more complex pathology. The disappearance of specific clinic-pathologic variants of vasculitis that are commonly encountered in practice was one important shortcoming of the 1994 classification. With advancing research and disclosure of a number of potential developmental and pathogenic interplayers provided an in-depth understanding of the disease. Scientific research illustrated that the vascular developmental patterns and the territorial distribution are major determinants of vessel wall reactivity to inflammation, endothelial antigenic cross talks, and response to inflammatory mediators. Vascular beds in different organs vary with respect to organ function in multiple aspects including morphology and function of the endothelial cells, intercellular junctions, the subendothelial matrix, the types of matrix components (including collagens, laminins, nidogens, fibronectin, vitronectin, and fibrillins), membrane proteins (adhesion molecules and Toll-like receptors—TLRs), and the pericytes that surround the endothelial cells. Such variations influence cell proliferation, migration, differentiation, transvascular passage of solutes and cellular diapedesis, chemotaxis, and tissue injury-response patterns. Microvascular diversities have been even seen within the same organ with the kidney featuring one good model [1–4].

In 2012, the Chapel Hill Consensus Conference went for revision of the 1994 classification to provide more precise classification of vasculitis with illustration of the different forms of vasculitis encountered in practice considering the nature of the pathology, the vessel size, and the etiology [5] **Figure 1**.

Definitions for vasculitides adopted by the 2012 International Chapel Hill Consensus Conference on the Nomenclature of Vasculitides (CHCC2012) [5, 6]:

I. *Large-vessel vasculitis* (*LVV*): vasculitis predominantly affecting large arteries (the aorta and its major branches); however, any size may be affected. It includes two main subtypes:

  a. *Takayasu arteritis* (*TAK*): granulomatous arteritis affecting the aorta and/or its major branches in patients younger than 50 years. The consensus retained the eponym "Takayasu" against the proposed non-eponymous term "early onset granulomatous aortitis/arteritis" being more effective than any alternative.

  b. *Giant cell arteritis* (*GCA*): granulomatous arteritis, usually affecting the aorta and/or its major branches, with a higher predilection for the branches of the carotid and vertebral arteries usually in patients older than 50 years and commonly associated with polymyalgia rheumatic. The disease often involves the temporal artery with the term "temporal arteritis" being commonly in use; however, not all patients with GCA have temporal artery involvement.

II. *Medium-vessel vasculitis* (*MVV*): vasculitis predominantly affecting medium-sized arteries defined as the main visceral arteries and their branches, and any size artery may be affected by the pathology. Inflammatory aneurysmal dilatations and arterial narrowing are common.

  a. *Polyarteritis nodosa* (*PAN*): necrotizing arteritis of the medium or small arteries or vasculitis in arterioles, capillaries, or venules, not associated with antineutrophil cytoplasmic antibodies (ANCAs).

  b. *Kawasaki disease* (*KD*): arteritis involving the medium- and small-sized arteries. The disease occurs in infants and young children presenting with mucocutaneous lymph node syndrome. Coronary arteritis remains a hallmark being frequently involved, while the aorta and large arteries may get involved.

III. *Small-vessel vasculitis* (*SVV*): vasculitis predominantly affecting small vessels defined as small intraparenchymal arteries, arterioles, capillaries, and venules. Similarly, medium arteries and veins may be affected.

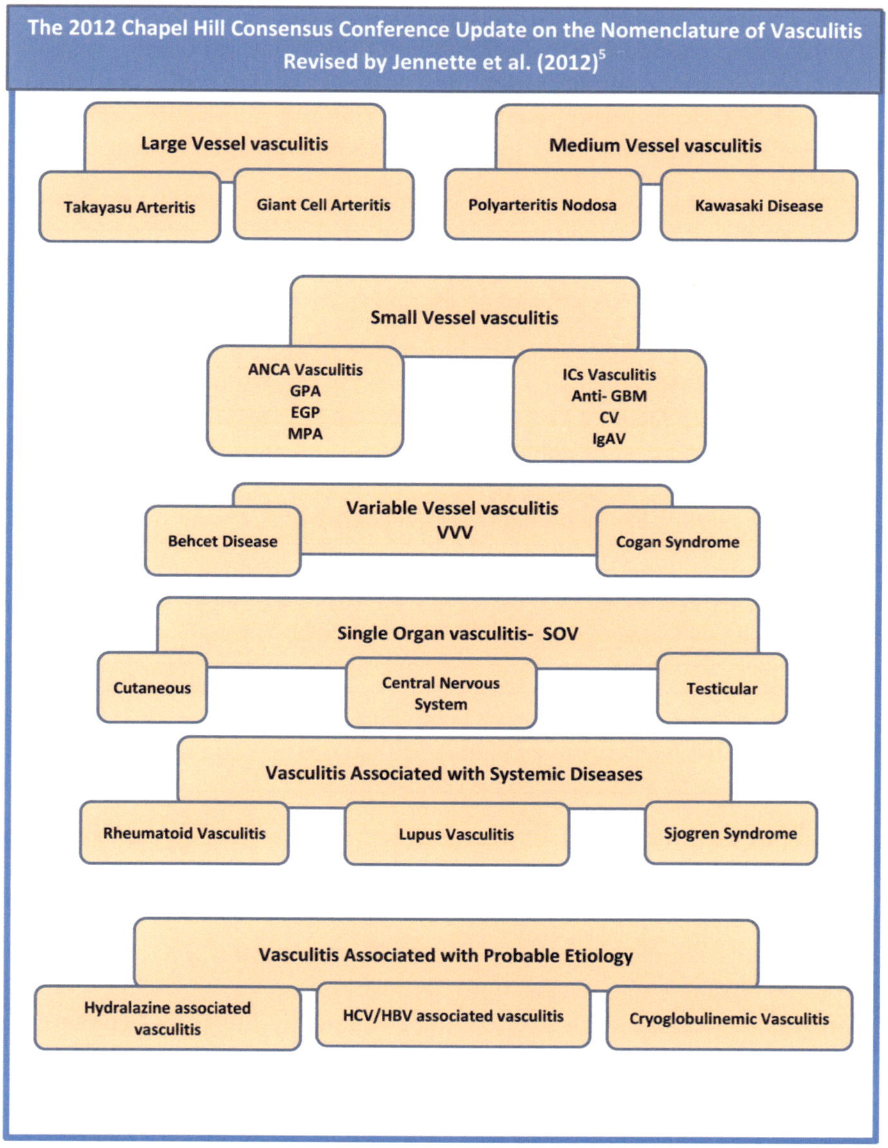

Figure 1. The 2012 Update of the Chapel Hill Consensus Conference on the Nomenclature and Classification of Vasculitides.

a. *ANCA-associated vasculitis* (*AAV*): necrotizing vasculitis, with few or no immune deposit, that is, pauci-immune necrotizing vasculitis, predominantly affecting the small vessels (i.e., capillaries, venules, arterioles, and small arteries), usually associated with antibodies to myeloperoxidase (MPO) or proteinase 3 (PR3) classified as either MPO-ANCA or PR3-ANCA, although not all the patients with this form of necrotizing vasculitis are ANCA positive.

1. *Microscopic polyangiitis* (*MPA*): necrotizing vasculitis, with few or no immune deposits, predominantly affecting small vessels (i.e., capillaries, venules, or arterioles). Necrotizing pauci-immune arteritis involving small- and medium-sized arteries and necrotizing glomerulonephritis and pulmonary capillaritis are frequent presentations, while granulomatous inflammation is absent.

2. *Granulomatosis with polyangiitis* (*Wegener's*) (*GPA*): necrotizing granulomatous vasculitis affecting predominantly from small to medium vessels (e.g., capillaries, venules, arterioles, arteries, and veins) usually involving the upper and lower respiratory tract. Necrotizing glomerulonephritis is common.

3. *Eosinophilic granulomatosis with polyangiitis* (*Churg-Strauss*) (*EGPA*): EGPA is an eosinophil-rich necrotizing granulomatous inflammation predominantly affecting from small to medium vessels often involving the respiratory tract and associated with asthma and eosinophilia. Nasal polyps are common. ANCA is more frequent when glomerulonephritis is present. The eponym "Churg-Strauss syndrome" was replaced by "EGPA" in part to achieve nomenclature symmetry with MPA and GPA.

b. *Immune complex vasculitis*: vasculitis predominantly affecting small vessels (i.e., capillaries, venules, arterioles, and small arteries) with moderate to marked immune complex deposits within vessel wall. Glomerulonephritis is frequent.

c. *Anti-glomerular basement membrane* (*anti-GBM*) *disease*: vasculitis affecting glomerular capillaries, pulmonary capillaries, or both, with GBM deposition of anti-GBM autoantibodies. Lung involvement causes pulmonary hemorrhage, and renal involvement causes glomerulonephritis with necrosis and crescents.

d. *Cryoglobulinemic vasculitis* (*CV*): vasculitis with immune deposits affecting small vessels (predominantly capillaries, venules, or arterioles) and associated with circulating cryoglobulins. Skin, glomeruli, and peripheral nerves are often involved.

e. *IgA vasculitis* (*Henoch-Schönlein*) (*IgAV*): vasculitis, with IgA1-dominant immune deposits, affecting small vessels (predominantly capillaries, venules, or arterioles). Skin, gastrointestinal tract, and joints are frequently involved. Glomerulonephritis indistinguishable from IgA nephropathy may occur.

f. *Hypocomplementemic urticarial vasculitis* (*HUV*) (*anti-C1q vasculitis*): vasculitis affecting small vessels (i.e., capillaries, venules, or arterioles) manifesting by urticaria and associated with hypocomplementemia and anti-C1q antibodies. Glomerulonephritis, arthritis, obstructive pulmonary disease, and ocular inflammation are common presentations.

IV. *Variable vessel vasculitis* (*VVV*): a form of vasculitis that can affect vessels of any size (small, medium, and large) and type (arteries, veins, and capillaries).

a. *Behcet's disease* (*BD*): vasculitis that can affect arteries or veins of variable calibers, characterized by recurrent oral and/or genital aphthous ulcers and accompanied by cutaneous, ocular, articular, gastrointestinal, and/or central nervous system inflammatory lesions. Small vessel vasculitis, thromboangiitis, thrombosis, arteritis, and arterial aneurysms may occur.

b. *Cogan's syndrome* (*CS*): Cogan's syndrome is a form of vasculitis that can affect vessels of variable sizes. The disease leads to arteritis (affecting small, medium, or large arteries), aortitis, aortic aneurysms, and aortic and mitral valvulitis. Clinically presents by ocular inflammatory lesions, including interstitial keratitis, uveitis, and episcleritis, and inner ear disease, including sensorineural hearing loss and vestibular dysfunction.

V. *Single-organ vasculitis* (*SOV*): vasculitis in arteries or veins of any size in a single organ that has no features that indicate that it is a limited expression of a systemic vasculitis. Vasculitis may be unifocal or multifocal/diffuse within the same organ. Usually defined in terms of the involved organ and vessel type, for example, cutaneous small vessel vasculitis, testicular arteritis, and central nervous system vasculitis. Some patients originally diagnosed as SOV may develop additional disease manifestations that warrant redefining the case as one of the systemic vasculitides, for example, cutaneous arteritis later becoming systemic polyarteritis nodosa, and so on.

VI. *Vasculitis associated with systemic disease*: vasculitis that is associated with and/or may be secondary to a systemic disease. The diagnosis should specify the systemic disease, for example, rheumatoid vasculitis, lupus vasculitis, and so on.

VII. *Vasculitis associated with probable etiology*: vasculitis that is associated with a probable specific etiology, for example, hydralazine-associated microscopic polyangiitis, hepatitis B virus-associated vasculitis, hepatitis C virus-associated cryoglobulinemic vasculitis, and so on.

In this book, the authors will provide and discuss an update on specific clinic-pathologic (**Figure 2**) subtypes of vasculitis including the pauci-immune vasculitis and immune

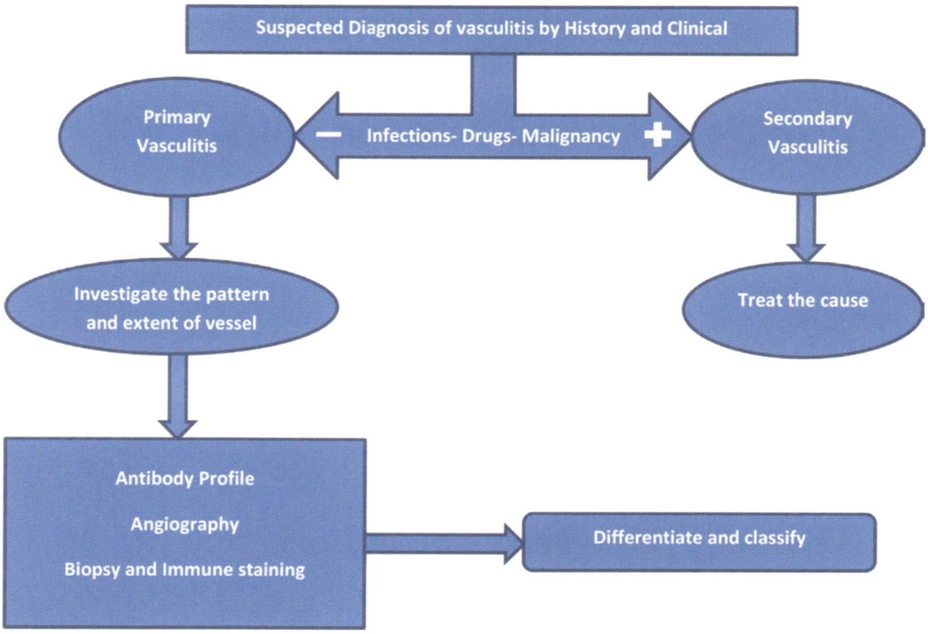

Figure 2. Algorithm for approaching diagnosis in vasculitis.

complex-mediated small vessel vasculitis with a special focus on renal disease among other vasculitis-related pathologies.

Author details

Reem Hamdy A. Mohammed

Address all correspondence to: rmhamdy@yahoo.com

Department of Rheumatology and Rehabilitation, Kasr Alaini School of Medicine, Cairo University, Egypt

References

[1] Hoffman G, Calabrese L. Vasculitis: Determinants of disease patterns. Nature Reviews Rheumatology. 2014;**10**:454-462

[2] Elefante E, Tripoli A, Ferro F, Baldini C. One year in review: Systemic vasculitis. Clinical and Experimental Rheumatology. 2016;**34**(Suppl. 97):S1-S6

[3] Jennette JC, Folk RJ, Andrassy K, et al. Nomenclature of systemic vasculitides: The proposal of an international consensus conference. Arthritis and Rheumatism. 1994;**37**: 187-192

[4] Falk RJ, Gross WL, Guillevin L, Hoffman GS, Jayne DR, Jennette JC, et al. American College of Rheumatology; American Society of Nephrology; European League Against Rheumatism. Granulomatosis with polyangiitis (Wegener's): An alternative name for Wegener's granulomatosis. Arthritis and Rheumatism. 2011 Apr;**63**(4):863-864

[5] Jennette JC, Folk RJ, Bacon K, et al. 2012 revised International Chapel Hill Consensus Conference nomenclature of vasculitides. Arthritis and Rheumatism. 2013;**65**:1-11

[6] Okazaki T, Shinagawa S, Mikage H. Vasculitis syndrome—Diagnosis and therapy. Journal of General and Family Medicine. 2017;**18**:72-78

Section 2

An update on Kidney Disease with Vasculitis

Chapter 2

Pauci-Immune Vasculitides with Kidney Involvement

Sophia Lionaki, Chrysanthi Skalioti,
Smaragdi Marinaki and John N. Boletis

Additional information is available at the end of the chapter

http://dx.doi.org/10.5772/intechopen.76175

Abstract

The clinical entity of pauci-immune vasculitis encompasses a group of diseases that may involve any organ system of the body and may be fatal if left untreated. This chapter will review these diseases, with a special interest in the clinical setting of kidney involvement. Small vessel vasculitides associated with the presence of antineutrophil cytoplasmic autoantibodies in the circulation will be the main part, since the vast majority of patients with histopathological proof of pauci-immune vasculitis are positive for these antibodies. Pauci-immune glomerulonephritis often manifests with rapidly deteriorating kidney function, while it may be accompanied by systemic necrotizing small vessel vasculitis such as microscopic polyangiitis, granulomatosis with polyangiitis, or eosinophilic granulomatosis with polyangiitis. Importantly, antineutrophil cytoplasmic autoantibody specificity has been shown to be associated with distinct clinical syndromes and different prognostic profiles among patients with pauci-immune vasculitis allowing easier recognition of the disease and long-term prognosis. Each of the clinical phenotypes will be described thoroughly with respect to the criteria required for establishment of diagnosis, the specific characteristics of renal and extrarenal histopathology, the clinical picture, the therapeutic management, and prognosis in short and long terms.

Keywords: pauci-immune, vasculitis, kidney involvement, rapidly progressive glomerulonephritis

1. Introduction

The principal characteristic of pauci-immune vasculitides is the paucity of staining for immunoglobulins in immunofluorescence, while they may occur as a renal-limited disease or as a component of systemic disease, i.e., necrotizing small vessel vasculitis [1, 2]. They affect small- and medium-sized vessels, and they represent the most common cause of crescentic glomerulonephritis, i.e., glomerulonephritis with 50% or more glomeruli being involved with crescents. The systemic vasculitides that may be accompanied by pauci-immune crescentic glomerulonephritis include three major clinical phenotypes: microscopic polyangiitis (MPA), granulomatosis with polyangiitis (GPA), and eosinophilic granulomatosis with polyangiitis (EGPA) [2]. An extremely big proportion (85–90%) of the patients with active untreated pauci-immune crescentic glomerulonephritis and vasculitis are positive for antineutrophil cytoplasmic antibodies (ANCA) [1], and therefore, the clinical entity is called ANCA-associated vasculitis. Distinct clinical syndromes and disease profiles have been associated with the type of ANCA. The classification of these diseases has been standardized by the Chapel Hill vasculitis nomenclature consensus conference in 1994 and revised in 2012. According to the current classification [3, 4] system for small vessel vasculitides, diagnostic definitions of ANCA-associated vasculitides include EGPA, which is characterized by the presence of asthma and eosinophilia, and necrotizing granulomatous inflammation is present [5], MPA is characterized by systemic necrotizing small vessel vasculitis with no evidence of granulomatous inflammation or asthma [5] and finally GPA if there is histopathological proof of necrotizing granulomatous inflammation or a clinical equivalent of it in any tissue. Moreover, patients with GPA are usually positive for C-ANCA (PR3-ANCA), patients with MPA are slightly more often positive for P-ANCA (MPO-ANCA), and patients with EGPA and renal-limited ANCA small vessel vasculitis have predominantly P-ANCA (MPO-ANCA) [1]. In some patients with pauci-immune vasculitis, conventional serologic assays fail to detect ANCA, although they present with the classic clinical and pathological characteristics of the disease. In this regard, recent advances in the field have shown that MPO-ANCA may react against a sole linear sequence in this group of patients [6].

This chapter will focus in pauci-immune vasculitides with kidney involvement, including the description of histopathological characteristics of renal and extrarenal lesions, epidemiology, pathogenesis, spectrum of clinical manifestations, definitions and diagnostic criteria of treatment response, and long-term outcomes. In addition, the current therapeutic options and prognostic factors resulting from recent advances in the understanding of correlations between laboratory and serological and clinical parameters will be reviewed.

2. Epidemiology

The incidence of pauci-immune glomerulonephritis has been shown to be higher in older patients, while distribution between genders appears equal [7–9]. In the United States specifically, it has been estimated in 3.1 cases/million/year, with the disease being significantly more frequent in Caucasians, males, and individuals older than 65 years, while 95% of cases were found ANCA positive at diagnosis [7, 10]. In Europe, the incidence has been reported is 1–2 cases in 100,000 [9, 11], with an increasing trend in recent years up to 2000 [12]. A potential explanation may be the increased awareness of these diseases among physicians and also the easier recognition of them after the introduction of ANCA testing. However, since the incidence has been shown relatively unchanged since the early 2000s, it is most probable that the increased physician awareness, following the introduction of ANCA testing in routine clinical practice, is the most possible reason [13]. Additionally, the incidence of GPA is higher than that of MPA in northern Europe, while MPA is predominant among cases of ANCA-associated vasculitis in southern Europe [13–15].

Likewise, the prevalence of ANCA-associated small vessel vasculitis has been estimated in 46–184 cases/million [13], with the rate increasing during the last two decades. Patient survival has been improved significantly during this period, as the treatment options are more effective and physicians are aware of the disease.

3. Genetic background

Genetic predisposition appears to play a critical role in ANCA vasculitis, as shown from several reports. A study in a multiethnic cohort of patients from the University of North Carolina at Chapel Hill (USA) showed that GPA is quite infrequent among African Americans [16] with the HLA-DRB1*15 allele being a risk factor for PR3-ANCA disease in this population [16]. It is probable that there is a variation of the HLA-DRB1*15 allele worldwide, which is also recognized in the variation of clinical phenotypes of the disease across different geographical areas. Furthermore, the overall incidence rate of ANCA disease was similar between Japan and Europe; GPA and PR3-ANCA vasculitis were shown to be much less common in Japan [13].

4. ANCA role in pathogenesis

ANCA are antibodies which are directed against proteins in the cytoplasmic granules of neutrophils and the lysosomes of monocytes. They were first reported by Dr. D. Davies in 1982 [17] and were subsequently correlated with Wegener's granulomatosis and microscopic polyangiitis [18, 19]. However, in 1988, it was shown that most of the patients with pauci-immune crescentic glomerulonephritis have ANCA in their circulation, irrespective of the coexistence or not of systemic vasculitis [8]. ANCA have been distinguished on the basis of indirect immunofluorescence microscopy; cytoplasmic, C-ANCA, or perinuclear, P-ANCA, depending on the given pattern, and by enzyme immunoassay; and anti-myeloperoxidase (MPO-ANCA) and anti-proteinase 3 (PR3-ANCA) depending on the antigen protein. More than 95% of cytoplasmic ANCA are PR3-ANCA, and more than 95% of perinuclear ANCA are MPO-ANCA. ANCA glomerulonephritis occurs as a renal-limited disease or as a component of systemic necrotizing small vessel vasculitis [8, 19, 20].

After the discovery of ANCA, great effort has been made in understanding the etiology and pathogenesis of these diseases in order to discover new therapies. A pathogenic role of ANCA has been demonstrated by clinical observations and experimental studies, i.e., in vitro studies, which reveal that both PR3 and MPO-ANCA IgG activate neutrophils that then release mediators of acute inflammation [21–24]. Accordingly, it has been found that neutrophils activated by ANCA IgG can kill cultured endothelial cells in some occasions while activation of neutrophils by ANCA causes integrin and cytokine receptor-mediated adherence to cultured endothelial cells and transmigration across the endothelial layer [1, 25] and conformational changes in β integrins, enhancing ligand binding. Furthermore, unregulated adhesion molecules in glomerular lesions, coming from kidney biopsy specimens of patients with ANCA-associated vasculitis, support the interaction of ANCA-activated neutrophils with vessels [26].

However, the most significant evidence that ANCA are involved in the pathogenesis of these diseases are provided by in vivo studies and specifically by a mouse model in which passive transfer of anti-MPO IgG (MPO-ANCA) or anti-MPO lymphocytes resulted in induction of glomerulonephritis. Xiao et al. developed a model in which intravenous administration of anti-MPO IgG into either immunocompetent mice, or Rag2−/− mice that have no functioning T or B cells, causes pauci-immune crescentic glomerulonephritis and small vessel vasculitis, remarkably similar to human disease. Within a period of 6 days after the injection, all mice developed glomerulonephritis identical with the human one, while some of them developed manifestations of systemic vasculitis, with leukocytoclastic angiitis, necrotizing arteritis, lung capillaritis, and necrotizing granulomatosis inflammation [1, 27–30]. Likewise, severe crescentic glomerulonephritis with systemic vasculitis can be caused by passive transfer of splenocytes from MPO−/− mice that have been immunized with murine MPO. The renal injury in this model is exacerbated by stimulation with LPS [29] and appears dependent on an intact alternative complement pathway and the presence of neutrophils [31]. Another model produced focal segmental pauci-immune glomerulonephritis and focal pulmonary capillaritis in rats by immunization with human MPO, which induced anti-MPO antibodies that cross react with human and rat MPO [32].

Importantly, there are patients who carry a clear clinical and histopathological diagnosis of pauci-immune necrotizing and crescentic glomerulonephritis and vasculitis, in whom negative tests for ANCA are coming out repetitively. This might lead to significant delays in establishing the correct diagnosis and initiating appropriate immunosuppressive treatment. Exploring this issue, a multicenter study recently reported the development of a novel assay to identify specific target epitopes for ANCA [6], a methodology, which led to the detection of MPO-ANCA in patients with ANCA-negative disease that reacted against a sole linear sequence. Autoantibodies against this specific epitope had certain pathogenic properties, as demonstrated by their capacity to activate neutrophils in vitro and to induce nephritis in mice. Interestingly, the researchers detected a fragment of ceruloplasmin in serum, which was eliminated in purified IgG, allowing detection of ANCA subsequently. Besides, patients with ANCA-negative small vessel vasculitis were found to have a restricted autoantibody response against the linear epitope on MPO (aa 447–459), which is the same one that was found to be associated with active disease in the MPO-ANCA-positive patients group and declined upon clinical remission [6]. The authors concluded that that epitope specificity defines pathogenicity [6].

5. Vasculitic manifestations and ANCA specificity

The antigen against which ANCA is directed, i.e., ANCA specificity, has been shown to be strongly associated with the clinical manifestations of the disease, including the affected organ systems and the histopathological findings, in patients with pauci-immune vasculitis. In this regard, patients with renal-limited disease, or any form of vasculitis without any radiological or histological proof of granulomas, have been shown more likely to have MPO-ANCA, while those with necrotizing granulomatous inflammation were shown to have a higher probability to have PR3-ANCA. This was captured in a study of 523 patients with biopsy-proven ANCA small vessel vasculitis, where the vast majority of patients with renal-limited disease had MPO-ANCA (81%), while almost all patients with bone destruction or saddle nose deformity had PR3-ANCA (94%) [33]. The relationship between PR3- or MPO-ANCA and the anatomic site of the vasculitic manifestation and/or the presence of granulomatous inflammation has been shown remarkable. When vasculitis is expanding from the renal parenchyma to the gastrointestinal or respiratory tract, MPO-ANCA is found less frequent, while PR3-ANCA constantly increases. In patients with histological proof of granuloma at any site, 79% were shown to have PR3-ANCA, and 21% were shown to have MPO-ANCA. Therefore, MPO- or PR3-ANCA are associated with clinically distinct vasculitic syndromes, a principle which is proven critical for the classification of ANCA small vessel vasculitis and in clinical practice. Importantly, this relationship has been confirmed by a genome-wide association study, which showed that the pathogenesis of ANCA small vessel vasculitis has a substantial genetic component, with clear genetic distinctions greatly associated with ANCA specificity [34].

6. Diagnosis of pauci-immune glomerulonephritis

Clinical or pathologic evidence of renal disease is seen in approximately 90% of patients with MPA, 80% of patients with GPA and 45% of patients with EGPA. Pauci-immune crescentic glomerulonephritis is typically associated with ANCA, since 80–90% of pauci-immune crescentic glomerulonephritis occurs in ANCA-positive patients [1, 2, 20, 35]. The clinical presentation of patients with pauci-immune glomerulonephritis includes a range of disease activity starting from asymptomatic hematuria to rapidly progressive glomerulonephritis. In most cases however, clinical presentation is characterized by an elevated serum creatinine in combination with active urine sediment, i.e., demonstrating dysmorphic erythrocyturia with or without red blood cell casts and various degrees of proteinuria [36]. Rapidly progressing glomerulonephritis is characterized by reduced glomerular filtration rate occurring in a few days or weeks which cannot be attributed to other causes of acute kidney injury. A kidney biopsy in such occasion reveals, as said earlier, fibrinoid necrosis along with crescent formation in more than 50% of the glomeruli [1]. Yet, a significant proportion of patients present with acute renal failure requiring dialysis at the time of disease diagnosis.

7. Extrarenal manifestations

Constitutional symptoms often precede or come with the actual onset of the disease and include low-grade fever, fatigue, weight loss, myalgias, and arthralgias [5, 37]. The vast majority of patients (94%) when asked reported a prodromal "flu-like syndrome" before the overt vasculitic syndrome [40]. Beyond this there is a wide range of extrarenal manifestations of vasculitis including involvement of any site of the body, such as the upper airways, the lungs, the gastrointestinal tract, the nerves, and the skin.

Disease of the ear, nose, and throat system, in different forms and degrees of severity, is present in 90% of patients with GPA [1, 38, 39]. Typical symptoms are nasal crusting and obstruction, bloody nasal discharge or epistaxis-related nasal mucosa ulceration, sinus pain with associated drainage, otitis media, and hearing loss. In patients with GPA, the vessels supplying the cartilage may be affected, and septal perforation may occur, while invading granulomas may cause destructive bone disease disrupting the anatomy of such patients. Saddle nose deformation due to collapse of the nasal structure and facial paralysis due to facial nerve entrapment may be seen, but the most dangerous complication of upper respiratory involvement is the inflammation of the trachea, especially in the subglottic region, because it may result in airway stenosis. Subglottic stenosis and destruction in the sinonasal anatomy represent characteristic manifestations of GPA. Lung involvement may manifest as necrotizing granulomatous inflammation or alveolar capillaritis and is typically demonstrated on radiographic studies as nodular opacities or alveolar infiltrates. Pulmonary nodules may cavitate, thus making disease management difficult; infections are superimposed. Capillaritis, arteritis, and granulomatous inflammation may cause hemoptysis or massive pulmonary hemorrhage, life-threatening conditions, which require immediate induction therapy. Among patients with biopsy-proven pauci-immune glomerulonephritis, 53% were found to have pulmonary involvement manifested as hemoptysis or massive hemorrhage which quickly became fatal in 50% of them [1, 37]. Involvement of the skin with palpable purpura and nodules occurs in as many as 25% of patients. Other skin lesions include erythematous macular lesions, papules, infarcts, and necrotic ulcers. Vasculitic lesions in the mucous membranes manifest as aphthous stomatitis or oral ulceration. Eye involvement includes conjunctivitis, episcleritis, blepharitis, keratitis, or acute visual loss or orbital mass. Approximately 30% of patients report symptoms of abdominal pain, gastritis, ischemic colitis, or pancreatitis due to involvement of the vessels in abdominal organs. Occasional infarction of the bowel with viscus perforation and polymicrobial sepsis may result in life-threatening phenomena. Cranial nerve palsy, sensory peripheral neuropathy, or mononeuritis multiplex may be seen. Peripheral neuropathy caused by vasculitis in epineurial arterioles and arteries occurs in approximately 30% of patients. Vessels in the central nervous system can also be affected leading to sudden onset of seizures, cerebrovascular events, and cognitive disorders. Besides, deep vein thrombosis may occur, more frequently among patients with ANCA-associated vasculitis than the general population or other autoimmune disorders [39–41]. Anti-plasminogen autoantibodies have been identified in patients with PR-3 ANCA glomerulonephritis, as a result of utilization of a peptide coded by the antisense RNA of the PRTN3 gene [41], and have been associated with such thrombotic phenomena.

The clinical phenotype of EGPA probably denotes a somewhat different disease, manifested by asthma, eosinophilia, and granulomatous inflammation in the lung. ANCA are positive in 70% of the patients, most commonly MPO-ANCA [36], and eosinophilia greater than 10% in the peripheral blood is found. Coronary arteritis and myocarditis are the main causes of morbidity and mortality, accounting for 50% of deaths. Renal disease is much less frequent and less severe in this disease category, while neuropathy and cardiac disease are more common.

However, recent advances in EGPA suggest that the majority of patients, who are ANCA positive, also have glomerulonephritis, while those lacking ANCA are more likely to have cardiac disease [42].

8. Histopathology

8.1. Renal histopathology

The hallmark histopathologic lesions of acute pauci-immune glomerulonephritis are crescents and fibrinoid necrosis (**Figure 1**), which are found at the same frequency, irrespective of the presence or absence of systemic vasculitis [2, 43]. A wide range of lesions in terms of activity and severity may be found, ranging from focal segmental fibrinoid necrosis affecting less than 10% of glomeruli to severe diffuse necrotizing and crescentic glomerulonephritis that may injure all glomeruli (**Figure 2**). Breaks in Bowman's capsule are frequent [44]. Another element, which may be found, although not disease specific, is periglomerular granulomatous inflammation [1]. ANCA-associated glomerulonephritis is by definition pauci-immune, which means that immunofluorescence microscopy reveals no staining or a low level of staining (less than +2, in the 0–4 scale) (**Figure 3**) [45]. In a significant number of patients, there is evidence for antecedent glomerular or tubulointerstitial injury, manifested by glomerular sclerosis, fibrocellular crescents, and interstitial fibrosis. These lesions may be found in different stages of activity or resolution depending on the status of the disease. Nearly 10% of biopsy specimens have necrotizing inflammation in small cortical arteries or vascular inflammation of the medullary vasa rectae (**Figure 4**), causing papillary necrosis if it is severe.

8.2. Extrarenal histopathology

The pathologic features of pauci-immune vasculitic lesions are identical in other organs as they are in the kidney. Consequently, leukocytoclastic angiitis affecting vasa recta is very

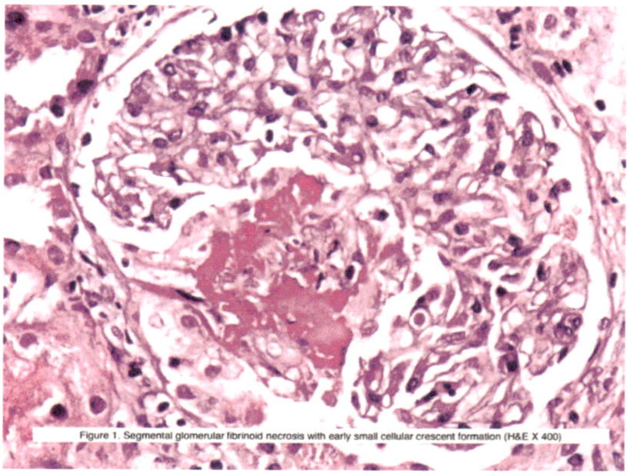

Figure 1. Segmental glomerular fibrinoid necrosis with early small cellular crescent formation (H&E 400×).

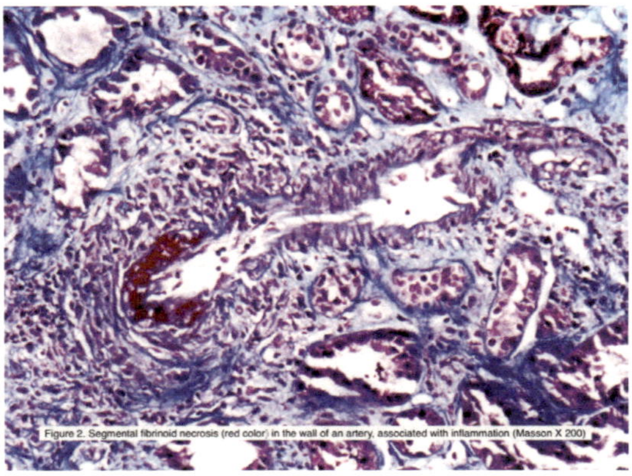

Figure 2. Segmental fibrinoid necrosis (red color) in the wall of an artery, associated with inflammation (Masson 200×).

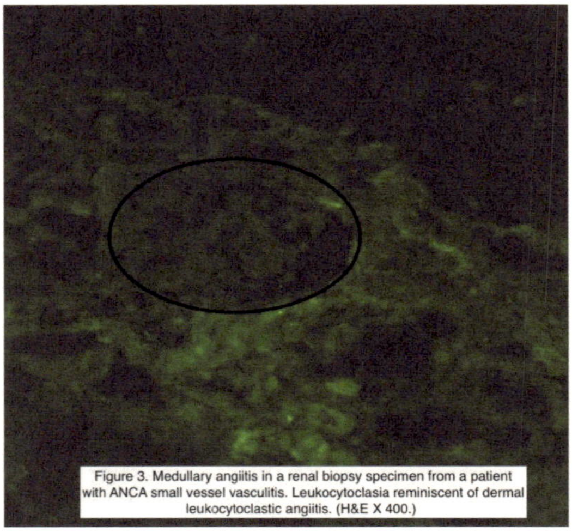

Figure 3. Medullary angiitis in a renal biopsy specimen from a patient with ANCA small vessel vasculitis. Leukocytoclasia reminiscent of dermal leukocytoclastic angiitis (H&E 400×).

similar to that in dermal venules, necrotizing capillaritis in glomeruli is identical to that in pulmonary capillaries, and necrotizing arteriolitis and arteritis in renal arteries are histologically indistinguishable from the necrotizing arteriolitis and arteritis in any site of the body, such as perineural arteritis causing peripheral neuropathy, gastrointestinal arteritis leading to focal ulceration and hemorrhage, and skeletal muscle arteritis leading to myalgias [1]. The histopathological proof of pauci-immune vasculitis prerequisites a paucity of staining for immunoglobulins [1] in order to confirm the diagnosis, and thus if glomerulonephritis is not present, a tissue biopsy at any site of active disease in any organ should be obtained.

The characteristic histological lesion in the pulmonary system in patients with MPA is capillaritis, while among patients with GPA, granulomatous inflammation may be seen as well. The necrotizing granulomatous inflammation may involve the upper and/or lower

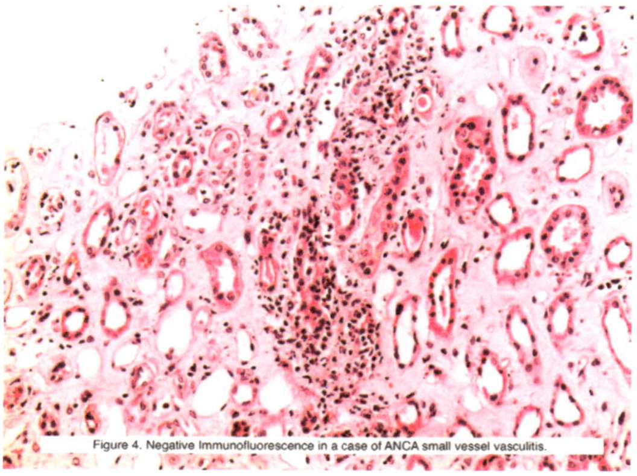

Figure 4. Negative immunofluorescence in a case of ANCA small vessel vasculitis.

respiratory system but may be found in any site, such as in the dermis and subcutaneous tissue. Granulomas are characterized histologically by an irregular central zone of necrosis that may have an amphophilic or bluish hue because of finely dispersed nuclear debris [1]. One major element of this lesion is epithelioid macrophages which may be numerous, but they do not have the compact arrangement seen in other occasions such as sarcoidosis [1]. Over time, extensive fibroblastic proliferation is usually seen, which ultimately may evolve into dense fibrotic scars. Nevertheless, for any specimen with necrotizing granulomatous inflammation, major non-vasculitic differential diagnostic considerations should be made, including myobacterial and fungal infections which need to be ruled out [1]. Conclusively, several sites of extrarenal involvement may be used to obtain a tissue biopsy, in order to have histopathological proof of the disease. A lung biopsy often requires an open or thoracoscopic lung procedure, while in a small proportion of patients, sufficient tissue for diagnosis can be obtained by transbronchial biopsy. Yet, the absence of granulomatous vasculitis on transbronchial specimens should not be considered adequate evidence to exclude the diagnosis of GPA [46]. A nasal biopsy is relatively easy and noninvasive, but its diagnostic power is limited by the high rate of false-negative results, probably related to the fact that the amount of tissue that can be removed is small. A positive lung biopsy is establishing the diagnosis in such cases and from one view precludes the need for a kidney biopsy in many cases; however, a renal biopsy is still indicated in patients who are diagnosed by lung biopsy, especially if they have severe or rapidly progressive renal involvement, in order to assess prognosis and plan immunosuppressive therapy in short and long term.

9. Definitions in relation to response to therapy

Diagnosis of active ANCA disease is followed by initiation of immunosuppressive therapy with the main goal being induction of remission, defined as stabilization or improvement of kidney function, measured by serum creatinine levels, resolution of hematuria, and all other organ-specific vasculitic symptoms [36]. However, some patients may not respond sufficiently, a phenomenon which is called "treatment resistance" and characterized by progressive decline in kidney function with persistent active urine sediment, or persistence or new appearance of any extrarenal vasculitic manifestations despite appropriate treatment. In addition, there are patients who initially responded to therapy in a manner that let them escape life-threatening or advanced organ damage, but it was not feasible for them to achieve complete obliteration of the pathogenic process and thus maintained a low grade of persistent activity known as "grumbling disease." Yet, patients achieving remission either complete or on therapy may or may not experience one or more disease relapses afterward. These are usually manifested as vasculitic signs or symptoms in any organ system, although relapses tend to affect the same organ systems as on initial presentation, with a new organ involvement reported only in 23% of patients [36].

10. Initial treatment

The gold standard of treatment in ANCA-associated vasculitis is the combination of corticosteroids with the cytotoxic agent cyclophosphamide [37, 47–50]. Glucocorticoids are given as intravenous pulses of methyl-prednisolone (7 mg/kg for 3 consecutive days) followed by oral prednisone (1 mg/kg for the first 4 weeks), reduced in a gradual and personalized manner over the next 3–5 months [2]. The protocol of treatment with cyclophosphamide in ANCA disease includes monthly pulses, given intravenously, starting at a dose of 0.5 g/m^2, subsequently increased up to 1 g/m^2, or orally at an initial dose of 2 mg/kg/day, always adjusted on the patient's leukocyte count. The duration of therapy with cyclophosphamide is usually 6–12 months, depending on patient's initial response [38, 47–51]. Both oral and intravenous schemes of cyclophosphamide have been proven equally effective in induction of remission [49], with the cumulative dose being significantly lower in the parenteral administration. In terms of achieved remission rates, a multivariate analysis showed superior results with the intravenous regimen without significant higher relapse rates [49]. Yet, a retrospective study showed [50] that the intravenous scheme of cyclophosphamide is associated with a higher risk of relapse, but this was not associated with increased rates of end-stage renal disease (ESRD), mortality, or long-term morbidity [50].

More recently, rituximab, a chimeric monoclonal antibody which is directed against the CD20 antigen of B lymphocytes, has also been used to induce remission in patients with ANCA-associated vasculitis, either in combination with steroids or cyclophosphamide and steroids [52]. A study authored by Jones et al. [52] compared rituximab with cyclophosphamide, as inductive therapy in patients with newly diagnosed ANCA-associated vasculitis with renal involvement, to a glucocorticoid regimen plus either rituximab with two intravenous cyclophosphamide pulses, or intravenous cyclophosphamide for 3–6 months followed by azathioprine. The scheme which contained rituximab, as part of therapy, was not superior to the standard one with intravenous cyclophosphamide (76 vs. 82%), with remission rates being high in both groups, while the rituximab regimen was not associated with fewer severe adverse events in the early phase [52]. Another study, which enrolled 197 ANCA-positive patients with either GPA or MPA, compared treatment with rituximab to treatment with oral cyclophosphamide for induction of remission. The rituximab-based regimen was shown more efficacious than the cyclophosphamide-based regimen for inducing remission of relapsing disease (67 vs. 42%, p = 0.01). Rituximab was also as effective as cyclophosphamide in the treatment of patients with renal or pulmonary involvement [52].

There are two clear indications which justify addition of plasma exchange in the inductive phase of treatment in ANCA-associated vasculitis: pulmonary hemorrhage and severe renal dysfunction at clinical presentation (serum creatinine is greater than 500 μmol/L). Pulmonary hemorrhage, either as isolated capillaritis, or as part of the pulmonary renal syndrome, may be a life-threatening condition leading to high mortality rates [1, 53, 54]. A retrospective study showed that the prompt institution of plasma exchange in addition to immunosuppressive therapy is 100% lifesaving [55] for these patients with diffuse pulmonary hemorrhage due to ANCA vasculitis, when compared to 50% historical controls. Furthermore, a randomized controlled study of 137 patients within the European Vasculitis Society (EUVAS) group with ANCA glomerulonephritis showed a clear benefit with the addition plasmapheresis to standard treatment in patients with severe renal impairments (serum creatinine >500 μmol/L). Specifically, addition of plasmapheresis was associated with a reduction in risk for progression to ESRD of 24% at 12 months and was also shown to be a positive predictor of dialysis independence at 1 year in patients with renal failure [54] (**Figure 5**).

Aggressive immunosuppressive therapy is warranted in patients with ANCA-associated small vessel vasculitis, since patient and renal survival have been shown very poor in untreated patients [38]. However, toxicity related to therapy is also problematic. For instance,

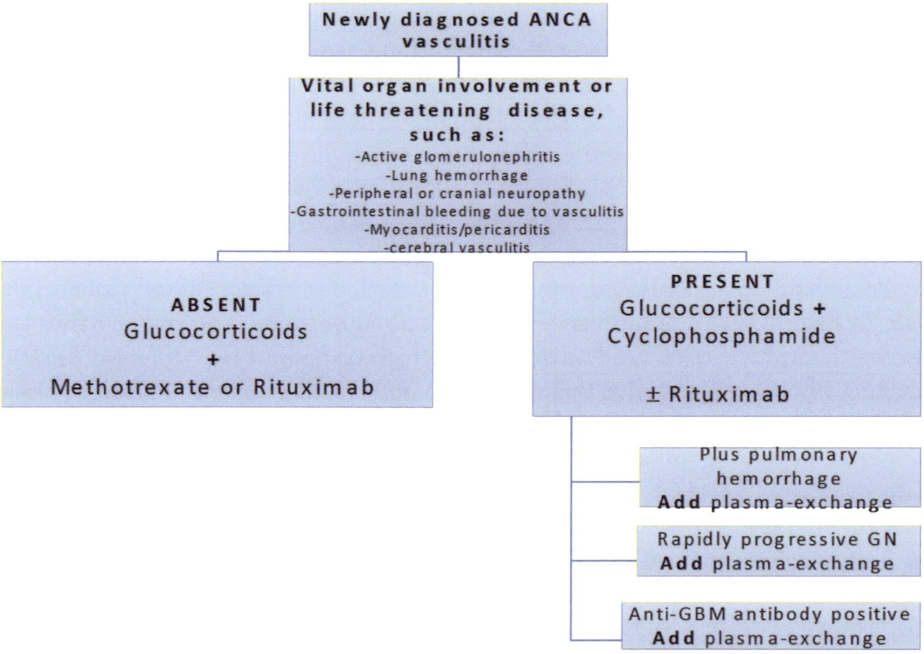

Figure 5. Algorithm to guide initial therapy for patients with newly diagnosed ANCA-associated vasculitis.

glucocorticoid therapy is associated with osteoporosis, glucose intolerance, and changes in body habitus in the long term, while life-threatening infections may occur during the acute phase. The frequency of severe infections is higher with the addition of cyclophosphamide. Moreover, therapy with cyclophosphamide has been associated with myelosuppression and hemorrhagic cystitis which occurs in 10% of patients. Bladder cancer has been estimated in 5% in 10 years and 16% in 15 years in patients treated with long-term oral cyclophosphamide. Myelodysplasia, lymphoma, skin cancer, and gonadal dysfunction are also associated with cyclophosphamide therapy [56]. Sufficient hydration and administration of 2-mercaptoethanesulfonate have been used in order to minimize urotoxicity.

Of note, although histopathological diagnosis is always desirable for patients with ANCA disease, we should underline that immunosuppressive treatment should be started empirically if the clinical suspicion for ANCA small vessel vasculitis is high and a tissue diagnosis cannot be obtained in a timely manner [18]. This is very important in order to avoid irreversible damage since these diseases often follow a rapidly progressive course with devastating consequences of the involved tissue.

11. Maintenance of remission

After achievement of remission, the disease course varies substantially among patients with ANCA small vessel vasculitis [10, 18]. Occurrence of relapse ranges from 30 to 50%. The majority of patients experience, either sustained long-term remission, or with one or more relapses occurring over time. Some patients continue having persistent, low-grade activity [10, 38]. Yet, evaluation of outcomes in patients in whom immunosuppressive therapy was discontinued after they attained remission showed similar rates of relapse compared to patients who remained on treatment for longer periods [10]. In the light of irreversible side effects related to therapy and relapse rates being comparable between long-term treated and not treated responders [10], optimal duration of immunosuppressive therapy should be decided on an individualized manner. In this regard, maintenance treatment is legitimate for patients who have a high rate of relapse, who have had a relapse already, or who maintain some disease activity despite full treatment. Undoubtedly, it is a challenge to select those patients in whom it is safe to discontinue therapy versus those who require remission maintenance therapy [10]. Recently, a prospective randomized trial, which compared two different durations of maintenance immunosuppressive therapy for the prevention of relapse in ANCA-associated vasculitis [55] showed that prolonged remission maintenance therapy with azathioprine/prednisolone, beyond 24 months after diagnosis, reduces relapse risk out to 48 months and improves renal survival. Nonetheless, the optimum duration of maintenance therapy depends on multiple factors. Another randomized controlled trial of patients with PR3-ANCA disease who remained ANCA positive at the time of stable remission, extending the duration of maintenance therapy with azathioprine from 1 year to 4 years (followed by taper), was not associated with a significant difference in relapse-free survival at 4 years [35, 57]. Finally, these results should not be extrapolated to other agents, especially since the optimal duration of maintenance therapy with rituximab has not been formally evaluated. A practical approach for clinicians is to use predictors of relapse, in order to be able to distinguish those patients who are at increased risk to relapse. Predictors of relapse among responders in ANCA-associated vasculitis have been shown to be PR3-ANCA seropositivity [33] and pulmonary and ear, nose, and throat involvement, each associated with an approximately two-fold increase in risk for relapse.

In terms of the agents which may be used, for maintenance of remission, conversion from cyclophosphamide to azathioprine at a dose of 2 mg/kg/day has been shown to be a safe choice with less toxicity [1, 56]. Furthermore, an open-label randomized controlled trial which was conducted in 156 patients from 42 European centers found that mycophenolate mofetil was less effective than azathioprine for maintaining remission, while adverse event rates were not different [56]. Employment of rituximab for the maintenance of remission in patients with ANCA vasculitis was tested in a study of 115 patients with GPA, MPA, or renal-limited disease after achievement of complete remission with cyclophosphamide and glucocorticoid [57]. Patients received either 500 mg of rituximab on days 0 and 14 and at months 6, 12, and 18 after study entry or daily azathioprine until month 22. In the rituximab group, more patients had sustained remission at month 28 than the azathioprine group, while the frequency of severe adverse events was similar between groups [58]. The antimicrobial agent trimethoprim-sulfamethoxazole has also been proven to prevent relapse in patients with GPA, by reducing the episodes of infections, probably by eliminating *Staphylococcus aureus* in the upper airways [59].

12. Management of persistent, refractory, or relapsing disease

Despite available options of treatment, some patients experience persistent symptoms or episodes of active inflammation that come up repentantly. In this regard, there are some choices which have been explored as potential alternatives [60–64] in order to treat the disease and minimize toxicity related to cytotoxic therapy in patients with ANCA-associated vasculitis. Among them, methotrexate combined with corticosteroids has been shown to lead to remission in 60–90% [60–62], but it was associated with an elevated rate of relapse [60–62]. Besides, yet, the use of methotrexate has been limited to patients with predominantly extrarenal manifestations of vasculitis and preserved renal function (serum creatinine <2.5 mg/dl). As a result, patients with signs of kidney involvement should not be treated with methotrexate. Mycophenolate mofetil is a safe and therapeutically beneficial alternative for patients with non-life-threatening, recurrent, or resistant ANCA vasculitis according to the results of a pilot study [64]. More recently, there are several reports of refractory disease which has been managed with rituximab, combined with steroids or cyclophosphamide or both, and ended up in remarkable improvement [65–67] or even complete remission.

13. Prognosis of patient and renal survival

The most important question of both patients and physicians in the case of ANCA-associated vasculitis is the issue of long-term prognosis, especially considering the relapsing and remitting course of this disease in association with the cumulative toxicity of therapy. The relative risk of death has been shown to be almost nine times greater in patients with MPA, who presented with lung hemorrhage, and four times greater in patients with cytoplasmic versus perinuclear ANCA [67] although the risk of lung hemorrhage was not different from ANCA pattern. The use of cyclophosphamide lowered the risk of death nearly six times, compared to steroid therapy alone [67]. Accordingly, long-term analysis of patients with GPA, who had received treatment with prednisone and cyclophosphamide, revealed that age over 50 years at diagnosis and lung or kidney involvement were associated with an almost fourfold increased risk for death [67]. The strongest predictors of long-term renal survival were found to be entry serum creatinine value, black race, and arterial sclerosis on renal biopsy [67]. Despite the certain finding that the higher the entry serum creatinine, the worse the long-term renal prognosis, no level of serum creatinine value could be determined beyond which treatment was futile, since 50% of the dialysis-dependent patients at onset recovered renal function permitting cessation of dialysis [67]. Taken all together, prompt institution of therapy remains the gold standard in these diseases. The risk for progression to ESRD after initial response to treatment in patients with ANCA glomerulonephritis was the change in GFR within 4 months of treatment. In this regard, after controlling for baseline creatinine level, type of treatment, and ANCA specificity, patients with a GFR decrease of 8 ml/min or greater were 5.6 times more likely to progress to ESRD than patients with stable GFR [10]. Relapse itself has also been shown to increase the probability of progression to ESRD by 4.7 times, with the related risk totally attributable to the recurrence of nephritis [10]. In patients with severe renal dysfunction due to ANCA glomerulonephritis, prognostic indicators of GFR after 12 months were shown to be age, the percentage of normal glomeruli, tubular atrophy, and intraepithelial infiltrates in the renal biopsy [51], while for those who were dialysis dependent at diagnosis, the probability for renal recovery was significantly increased with the addition of plasmapheresis [54].

Prediction of treatment resistance has been studied in a large cohort of patients with ANCA-associated vasculitis [67], recruited by kidney disease, which showed that 23% of the 334 treated patients became refractory to standard therapy. Most of them ended up to ESRD in median of 2 months after initiation of therapy. Female sex, black ethnicity, and severity of renal involvement were identified as predictors of treatment resistance. The risk of treatment resistance increased 1.28 times for each serum creatinine elevation of 100 μmol/L (1.13 mg/dl). Nonetheless, these rates have not been estimated with the newer agents and especially after the introduction of rituximab in the treatment of these diseases. Typically, these patients had a relapsing and remitting course not recognized by their primary care provider, leading to advanced glomerular and interstitial scarring at the time of diagnosis [67].

In conclusion, pauci-immune vasculitides, despite the substantial progress which has been achieved in the field of pathogenesis and treatment, remain a group of diseases with significant morbidity and mortality, related to the disease itself and the toxicity coming from therapy. Renal involvement is one of the most threatening aspects of this disease, especially considering the side effects related to renal insufficiency and chronic dialysis, in the case of extended irreversible damage of the renal tissue. Speed in diagnosis and prompt institution of appropriate immunosuppressive treatment endure the key of avoiding such outcome.

http://dx.doi.org/10.5772/intechopen.76175

Acknowledgements

We thank our renal pathologists Drs. Chara Gakiopoulou and George Liapis, for providing high-quality pictures showing pauci-immune glomerulonephritis.

A minor part of this document is taken from our previous work *The Prevalence and Management of Pauci-Immune Glomerulonephritis and Vasculitis in Western Countries* https://content.karger.com/Article/FullText/442062.

Conflict of interest

The authors have nothing to declare.

Author details

Sophia Lionaki*, Chrysanthi Skalioti, Smaragdi Marinaki and John N. Boletis

*Address all correspondence to: sofia.lionaki@gmail.com

Faculty of Medicine, Laiko Hospital, National and Kapodistrian University of Athens, Greece

References

[1] Jennette JC, Thomas DB. Pauci-immune and antineutrophil cytoplasmic autoantibody-mediated crescentic glomerulonephritis and vasculitis. In: Jennette JC, Olson JL, Schwartz MM, Silva FG, editors. Heptinstall's Pathology of the Kidney. Philadelphia: Lippincott, Williams & Wilkins; 2007. pp. 642-673

[2] Couser WG. Rapidly progressive glomerulonephritis: Classification, pathogenetic mechanisms, and therapy. American Journal of Kidney Diseases. 1988;**11**:449-464

[3] Jennette JC, Falk RJ, Andrassy K, et al. Nomenclature of systemic vasculitides. Proposal of an international consensus conference. Arthritis & Rheumatology. 1994;**37**:187-192

[4] Jennette JC, Falk RJ, Bacon PA, et al. 2012 revised international Chapel Hill consensus conference nomenclature of vasculitides. Arthritis and Rheumatism. 2013;**65**(1):1-11

[5] Jennette JC, Falk RJ. Small-vessel vasculitis. The New England Journal of Medicine. 1997; **337**:1512-1523

[6] Roth AJ, Ooi JD, Hess JJ, et al. Epitope specificity determines pathogenicity and detectability in ANCA-associated vasculitis. The Journal of Clinical Investigation. 2013;**123**(4): 1773-1783

[7] Jennette JC, Falk RJ. Clinical and pathological classification of ANCA-associated vasculitis: What are the controversies? Clinical and Experimental Immunology. 1995;**101**(Suppl 1): 18-22

[8] Falk RJ. ANCA-associated renal disease. Kidney International. 1990;**38**:998-1010

[9] Pettersson EE, Sundelin B, Heigl Z. Incidence and outcome of pauci-immune necrotizing and crescentic glomerulonephritis in adults. Clinical Nephrology. 1995;**43**:141-149

[10] Hogan SL, Falk RJ, Chin H, et al. Predictors of relapse and treatment resistance in anti-neutrophil cytoplasmic antibody-associated small-vessel vasculitis. Annals of Internal Medicine. 2005;**143**:621-631

[11] Savage CO, Harper L, Adu D. Primary systemic vasculitis. Lancet. 1997;**349**:553-558

[12] Knight A, Ekbom A, Brandt L, et al. Increasing incidence of Wegener's granulomatosis in Sweden, 1975-2001. The Journal of Rheumatology. 2006;**33**:2060-2063

[13] Watts RA, Mahr A, Mohammad AJ, et al. Classification, epidemiology and clinical subgrouping of antineutrophil cytoplasmic antibody (ANCA)-associated vasculitis. Nephrology, Dialysis, Transplantation. 2015;**30**(Suppl 1):i14-i22

[14] Haugeberg G, Bie R, Bendvold A, et al. Primary vasculitis in a Norwegian community hospital: A retrospective study. Clinical Rheumatology. 1998;**17**(5):364-368

[15] Watts RA, Lane SE, Bentham G, et al. Epidemiology of systemic vasculitis: A ten-year study in the United Kingdom. Arthritis and Rheumatism. 2000;**43**(2):414-419

[16] Cao Y, Schmitz JL, Yang J, et al. DRB1*15 allele is a risk factor for PR3-ANCA disease in African Americans. Journal of the American Society of Nephrology. 2011;**22**(6):1161-1167

[17] Davies DJ, Moran JE, Niall JF, et al. Segmental necrotising glomerulonephritis with anti-neutrophil antibody: Possible arbovirus aetiology? British Medical Journal. 1982;**285**:606

[18] Van Der Woude FJ, Rasmussen N, Lobatto S, et al. Autoantibodies against neutrophils and monocytes: Tool for diagnosis and marker of disease activity in Wegener's granulomatosis. Lancet. 1985;**1**:425-429

[19] Falk RJ, Jennette JC. Anti-neutrophil cytoplasmic auto-antibodies with specificity for myeloperoxidase in patients with systemic vasculitis and idiopathic necrotizing and crescentic glomerulonephritis. The New England Journal of Medicine. 1988;**318**:1651-1657

[20] Jennette JC, Thomas DB. Crescentic glomerulonephritis. Nephrology, Dialysis, Transplantation. 2001;**16**(Suppl 6):80-82

[21] Falk RJ, Terrell RS, Charles LA, Jennette JC. Anti-neutrophil cytoplasmic autoantibodies induce neutrophils to degranulate and produce oxygen radicals in vitro. Proceedings of the National Academy of Sciences of the United States of America. 1990;**87**:4115-4119

[22] Schreiber A, Busjahn A, Luft FC, et al. Membrane expression of proteinase 3 is genetically determined. Journal of the American Society of Nephrology. 2003;**14**:68-75

[23] Schreiber A, Luft FC, Kettritz R. Membrane proteinase 3 expression and ANCA-induced neutrophil activation. Kidney International. 2004;**65**:2172-2183

[24] Charles LA, Caldas ML, Falk RJ, et al. Antibodies against granule proteins activate neutrophils in vitro. Journal of Leukocyte Biology. 1991;**50**:539-546

[25] Radford DJ, Luu NT, Hewins P, et al. Antineutrophil cytoplasmic antibodies stabilize adhesion and promote migration of flowing neutrophils on endothelial cells. Arthritis and Rheumatism. 2001;**44**:2851-2861

[26] Moon KC, Park SY, Kim HW, et al. Expression of intercellular adhesion molecule-1 and vascular cell adhesion molecule-1 in human crescentic glomerulonephritis. Histopathology. 2002;**41**:158-165

[27] Xiao H, Heeringa P, Hu P, et al. Antineutrophil cytoplasmic autoantibodies specific for myeloperoxidase cause glomerulonephritis and vasculitis in mice. The Journal of Clinical Investigation. 2002;**110**:955-963

[28] Xiao H, Heeringa P, Liu Z, et al. The role of neutrophils in the induction of glomerulonephritis by anti-myeloperoxidase antibodies. The American Journal of Pathology. 2005;**167**:39-45

[29] Huugen D, Xiao H, Falk RJ, et al. Aggravation of anti-myeloperoxidase antibody-induced glomerulonephritis by bacterial lipopolysaccharide: Role of tumor necrosis factor-alpha. The American Journal of Pathology. 2005;**167**:47-58

[30] Jennette JC, Xiao H, Falk RJ. Pathogenesis of vascular inflammation by anti-neutrophil cytoplasmic antibodies. Journal of the American Society of Nephrology. 2006;**17**:1235-1242

[31] Xiao H, Schreiber A, Heeringa P, et al. Alternative complement pathway in the pathogenesis of disease mediated by anti-neutrophil cytoplasmic autoantibodies. The American Journal of Pathology. 2007;**170**:52-64

[32] Little MA, Smyth CL, Yadav R, et al. Antineutrophil cytoplasm antibodies directed against myeloperoxidase augment leukocyte-microvascular interactions in vivo. Blood. 2005;**106**:2050-2058

[33] Lionaki S, Blyth ER, Hogan SL, et al. Classification of antineutrophil cytoplasmic autoantibody vasculitides: The role of antineutrophil cytoplasmic autoantibody specificity for myeloperoxidase or proteinase 3 in disease recognition and prognosis. Arthritis and Rheumatism. 2012;**64**(10):3452-3462

[34] Lyons PA, Rayner TF, Trivedi S, et al. Genetically distinct subsets within ANCA-associated vasculitis. New England Journal of Medicine. 2012;**367**(3):214-223

[35] Jennette JC, Falk RJ. Pathogenesis of the vascular and glomerular damage in ANCA-positive vasculitis. Nephrology, Dialysis, Transplantation. 1998;**13**(Suppl 1):16-20

[36] Nachman PH, Hogan SL, Jennette JC, et al. Treatment response and relapse in antineutrophil cytoplasmic autoantibody-associated microscopic polyangiitis and glomerulonephritis. Journal of the American Society of Nephrology. 1996;**7**:33-39

[37] Falk RJ, Hogan S, Carey TS, Jennette JC. Clinical course of anti-neutrophil cytoplasmic autoantibody-associated glomerulonephritis and systemic vasculitis. The glomerular disease collaborative network. Annals of Internal Medicine. 1990;**113**:656-663

[38] Hoffman GS, Kerr GS, Leavitt RY, et al. Wegener granulomatosis: An analysis of 158 patients [see comments]. Annals of Internal Medicine. 1992;**116**:488-498

[39] Merkel P, Lo G, Holbrook J, et al. Thromboembolism—another threat to the polymorbid patient with vasculitis?: High incidence of venous thrombotic events among patients with Wegener granulomatosis: The Wegener's Clinical Occurrence of Thrombosis (WeCLOT) Study. Ann Intern Med 2005; 142: 620-626, 2005. Journal of the American Society of Nephrology. 2005;**16**:1871-1877

[40] Weidner S, Hafezi-Rachti S, Rupprecht HD. Thromboembolic events as a complication of antineutrophil cytoplasmic antibody-associated vasculitis. Arthritis and Rheumatism. 2006;**55**:146-149

[41] Bautz DJ, Lionaki S, Yang JJ, et al. The search for complementary PR3 proteins identified plasminogen as an autoantigen in PR3-ANCA disease. Journal of the American Society of Nephrology. 2006;**85A**:17

[42] Falk RJ, Hoffman GS. Controversies in small vessel vasculitis-comparing the rheumatology and nephrology views. Current Opinion in Rheumatology. 2007;**19**:1-9

[43] D'Agati V, Chander P, Nash M, Mancilla-Jimenez R. Idiopathic microscopic polyarteritis nodosa: Ultrastructural observations on the renal vascular and glomerular lesions. American Journal of Kidney Diseases. 1986;**7**:95-110

[44] Ferrario F, Tadros MT, Napodano P, Sinico RA, Fellin G, D'Amico G. Critical re-evaluation of 41 cases of "idiopathic" crescentic glomerulonephritis. Clinical Nephrology. 1994; **41**:1-9

[45] Harris AA, Falk RJ, Jennette JC. Crescentic glomerulonephritis with a paucity of glomerular immunoglobulin localization. American Journal of Kidney Diseases. 1998;**32**:179-184

[46] Schnabel A, Holl-Ulrich K, Dalhoff K, et al. Efficacy of transbronchial biopsy in pulmonary vasculitides. The European Respiratory Journal. 1997;**10**(12):2738-2743

[47] Fauci AS, Haynes BF, Katz P, Wolff SM. Wegener's granulomatosis: Prospective clinical and therapeutic experience with 85 patients for 21 years. Annals of Internal Medicine. 1983;**98**:76-85

[48] Novack SN, Pearson CM. Cyclophosphamide therapy in Wegener's granulomatosis. The New England Journal of Medicine. 1971;**284**:938-942

[49] de Groot K, Jayne DR, Tesar V, Savage CO. European, multicenter randomised controlled trial of daily oral versus pulse cyclophosphamide for induction of remission in ANCA-associated systemic vasculitis for the European Vasculitis Study Group. Annals of Internal Medicine 2009;**150**(10):670-680

[50] Harper L, Morgan MD, Walsh M, et al. Pulse versus daily oral cyclophosphamide for induction of remission in ANCA-associated vasculitis: Long-term follow-up. Annals of the Rheumatic Diseases. 2012;**71**(6):955-960

[51] de Lind van Wijngaarden RA, Hauer HA, Wolterbeek R, et al. Clinical and histologic determinants of renal outcome in ANCA-associated vasculitis: A prospective analysis of 100 patients with severe renal involvement. Journal of the American Society of Nephrology. 2006;**17**:2264-2274

[52] Jones RB, Tervaert JW, Hauser T, et al. European Vasculitis Study Group. Rituximab versus cyclophosphamide in ANCA-associated renal vasculitis. The New England Journal of Medicine. 2010;**363**(3):211-220

[53] Klemmer PJ, Chalermskulrat W, Reif MS, et al. Plasmapheresis therapy for diffuse alveolar hemorrhage in patients with small-vessel vasculitis. American Journal of Kidney Diseases. 2003;**42**:1149-1153

[54] Jayne DR, Gaskin G, Rasmussen N, et al. Randomized trial of plasma exchange or high-dosage methylprednisolone as adjunctive therapy for severe renal vasculitis. Journal of the American Society of Nephrology. 2007;**18**:2180-2188

[55] Karras A, Pagnoux C, Haubitz M, Groot K, Puechal X, Tervaert JWC, Segelmark M, Guillevin L, Jayne D. European Vasculitis Society. Randomised controlled trial of prolonged treatment in the remission phase of ANCA-associated vasculitis. Annals of the Rheumatic Diseases. 2017;**76**(10):1662-1668

[56] Hiemstra TF, Walsh M, Mahr A, et al. European Vasculitis Study Group (EUVAS). Mycophenolate mofetil vs azathioprine for remission maintenance in antineutrophil cytoplasmic antibody-associated vasculitis: A randomized controlled trial. JAMA. 2010; **304**(21):2381-2388

[57] Sanders JSF, de Joode AAE, De Sevaux RG, et al. Extended versus standard azathioprine maintenance therapy in newly diagnosed proteinase-3 anti-neutrophil cytoplasmic antibody-associated vasculitis patients who remain cytoplasmic anti-neutrophil cytoplasmic antibody-positive after induction of remission: A randomized clinical trial. Nephrology Dialysis Transplantation. 2016;**31**:1453-1459

[58] Jayne D, Rasmussen N, Andrassy K, et al. A randomized trial of maintenance therapy for vasculitis associated with antineutrophil cytoplasmic autoantibodies. The New England Journal of Medicine. 2003;**349**:36-44

[59] Guillevin L, Pagnoux C, Karras A, et al. French Vasculitis Study Group. Rituximab versus azathioprine for maintenance in ANCA-associated vasculitis. The New England Journal of Medicine. 2014;**371**(19):1771-1780

[60] Stegeman CA, Tervaert JW, De Jong PE, et al. Trimethoprim-sulfamethoxazole (co-trimoxazole) for the prevention of relapses of Wegener's granulomatosis. Dutch Co-Trimoxazole Wegener Study Group. New England Journal of Medicine. 1996;**335**:16-20

[61] Langford CA, Talar-Williams C, Barron KS, et al. A staged approach to the treatment of Wegener's granulomatosis: Induction of remission with glucocorticoids and daily cyclophosphamide switching to methotrexate for remission maintenance. Arthritis and Rheumatism. 1999;**42**:2666-2673

[62] Langford CA, Talar W, Sneller MC. Use of methotrexate and glucocorticoids in the treatment of Wegener's granulomatosis. Long-term renal outcome in patients with glomerulonephritis. Arthritis and Rheumatism. 2000;**43**:1836-1840

[63] Furst DE. Practical clinical pharmacology and drug interactions of low-dose methotrexate therapy in rheumatoid arthritis. British Journal of Rheumatology. 1995;**34**(Suppl 2):20-25

[64] Joy MS, Hogan SL, Jennette JC, et al. A pilot study using mycophenolate mofetil in relapsing or resistant ANCA small vessel vasculitis. Nephrology, Dialysis, Transplantation. DOI: 10.1093/ndt/gfi117

[65] McGregor JG, Hogan SL, Kotzen ES, et al. Rituximab as an immunosuppressant in antineutrophil cytoplasmic antibody-associated vasculitis. Nephrology, Dialysis, Transplantation. 2015;(Suppl 1):i123-i131

[66] Jones RB, Ferraro AJ, Chaudhry AN, Brogan P, Salama AD, Smith KG, Savage CO, Jayne DR. A multicenter survey of rituximab therapy for refractory antineutrophil cytoplasmic antibody-associated vasculitis. Arthritis and Rheumatism. 2009;**60**(7):2156-2168

[67] Hogan SL, Nachman PH, Wilkman AS, et al. Prognostic markers in patients with antineutrophil cytoplasmic autoantibody-associated microscopic polyangiitis and glomerulonephritis. Journal of the American Society of Nephrology. 1996;**7**:23-32

Chapter 3

Immune Complex Small-Vessel Vasculitis with Kidney Involvement

Smaragdi Marinaki, Chrysanthi Skalioti,
Sophia Lionaki and John N. Boletis

Additional information is available at the end of the chapter

http://dx.doi.org/10.5772/intechopen.77226

Abstract

The term immune complex small-vessel vasculitis encompasses anti-glomerular basement membrane disease, cryoglobulinemic vasculitis, IgA vasculitis and hypocomplementemic urticarial vasculitis. These disorders affect predominantly small vessels, and renal involvement is frequent. In this chapter, we shall discuss thoroughly anti-GBM disease, cryoglobulinemic and IgA vasculitis with respect to the criteria required for the establishment of diagnosis, the specific characteristics of renal histopathology, the clinical picture, prognosis, and therapeutic management.

Keywords: vasculitides, immune complex, immunoglobulin A (IgA) vasculitis, cryoglobulinemia, anti-glomerular basement membrane disease

1. Introduction

Immune complex small-vessel vasculitis (SVV) refers to vasculitis, which is characterized by the deposition of immunoglobulin and/or complement on the vessel wall. It affects predominantly small vessels, and renal involvement is common. According to the Chapel Hill consensus conference nomenclature of vasculitides [1], disorders included in the group of immune complex SVV are anti-glomerular basement membrane (anti-GBM) disease, cryoglobulinemic vasculitis (CV), IgA vasculitis (IgAV), and hypocomplementemic urticarial vasculitis.

Anti-GBM disease is a vasculitis, which affects glomerular and/or pulmonary capillaries. It is caused by autoantibodies against the basement membrane. Renal involvement typically causes acute or rapidly progressive glomerulonephritis.

Cryoglobulinemic vasculitis is characterized by the presence of cryoglobulins, which are immunoglobulins or immune complexes that precipitate in the cold and dissolve upon rewarming. Common sites of deposition are the skin, the joints, the peripheral nerves, and the kidneys. The main etiological factors are chronic viral infections, particularly autoimmune disorders and B-cell lymphoproliferative disorders.

IgA vasculitis is a systemic vasculitis characterized by the deposition of IgA1-dominant immune complexes. It affects predominantly the skin, the joints, and the gastrointestinal tract. Renal involvement with glomerular hematuria and mild proteinuria may be observed.

2. Anti-glomerular basement membrane disease

2.1. Introduction

Anti-glomerular basement membrane (anti-GBM) disease, also known as Goodpasture's syndrome, is an immune complex small-vessel vasculitis first identified by Dr. Ernest Goodpasture in 1919 [1, 2]. It is characterized by autoantibodies directed against the alpha-3 chain of type IV collagen of the glomerular and alveolar basement membrane. In 1951, Krakower and Greenspon discovered the antigenic properties of the glomerular basement membrane (GBM) [3], whereas, in 1967 Lerner, Glassock and Dixon found that autoantibodies eluted from kidneys with acute glomerulonephritis produce the disease in animal models [4]. Patients typically present with glomerulonephritis alone or in association with alveolar hemorrhage that can be life threatening.

2.2. Epidemiology

Anti-GBM disease is rare. The annual incidence is estimated to be about 0.5–1 cases per million inhabitants in Europe [5, 6]. The White race is affected more commonly than the Black race. Age distribution is bimodal, with a peak incidence in the third and seventh decades. A slight male predominance is recorded in the younger age group and a female predominance in the older [7].

2.3. Pathogenesis

Exposure to an exogenous stimulus leads to autoantibody production and circulation of antibodies, which are directed against an antigen of the glomerular basement membrane (GBM). This antigen has been identified as a particular region of the NC1 domain of the $\alpha3$ chain of type IV collagen.

Type IV Collagen is the main constituent of most basement membranes and is encoded by six genes (COL4A1-A6) each for six distinct α chains ($\alpha1$(IV) to $\alpha6$(IV)), which are selectively expressed in membranes of different organs through embryonic development. This selectivity explains the specific lung and renal involvement in Goodpasture's disease, since $\alpha3$IV collagen is expressed primarily in the GBM of the glomeruli and the pulmonary alveoli [8].

Each α chain consists of three domains: a short 7C domain at the N-terminal, a long collagenous domain in the middle, and a noncollagenous domain (NC1) at the C-terminal. During development, the six α chains form three sets of triple helical molecules called promoters:

$\alpha1\alpha1\alpha2$(IV), $\alpha3\alpha4\alpha5$(IV) and $\alpha5\alpha5\alpha6$(IV). These promoters subsequently form three-dimensional organized networks consisting of only three sets of hexamers: $\alpha1\alpha1\alpha2$ (IV)-$\alpha1\alpha1\alpha2$(IV), $\alpha3\alpha4\alpha5$(IV)-$\alpha3\alpha4\alpha5$(IV) and $\alpha1\alpha1\alpha2$(IV)-$\alpha5\alpha5\alpha6$(IV).

The autoantigen in anti-GBM is the α3NC1 domain which is located in the network of $\alpha3\alpha4\alpha5$(IV)-$\alpha3\alpha4\alpha5$(IV) hexamers. Two major antigenic epitopes E_A and E_B in the α3NC1 domain of the hexamer have been identified as targets for the autoantibodies [9, 10].

These epitopes are hidden and are only accessible to the autoantibodies after dissociation of the hexamer as a result of oxidative stress. This could explain the initiation of anti-GBM after an extrinsic insulting event as, for example, after a respiratory tract infection or after urinary tract obstruction or lithotripsy [11].

Anti-GBM autoantibodies are most often of the IgG class (usually IgG1 or 2 subclass) and rarely IgA. The pathogenicity of the autoantibodies has been demonstrated by induction of the disease after passive transfer of circulating or tissue autoantibodies in animal models. The high and rapid binding affinity to alveolar and glomerular capillary basement membranes is consistent with the fulminant disease course though variable pathogenicity according to autoantibody titers, different IgG subclass and epitope specificity has also been reported [12, 13].

Besides autoantibody production, there is growing evidence for the contribution of autoreactive T cells to the pathogenesis of anti-GBM. In some instances, autoantibodies alone are not sufficient to induce disease. Furthermore, T cells with reactivity against the α3NC1 antigen have been isolated from patients with the disease. In animal models, it has been demonstrated that CD4+ T cells specific for the Col4α3NC1 epitope can target the autoantigen and induce glomerular injury in the absence of autoantibodies, suggesting a direct causative role of T cells [9, 14].

2.3.1. Genetic susceptibility

The susceptibility to the development of the disease is genetically determined and restricted by the major histocompatibility complex (MHC): HLA-DR15 and HLA-DR4 haplotypes increase susceptibility while HLA-DR1 and HLA-DR7 seem to be protective [8, 15].

Moreover, anti-GBM autoantibodies occur after kidney transplantation in patients with hereditary nephritis (X-linked Alport's syndrome). This can be explained by the genetically defective organization of the α chains of type IV collagen. The genetic defect in hereditary nephritis results in the absence of $\alpha3\alpha4\alpha5$ (IV)-$\alpha3\alpha4\alpha5$(IV) hexamers and the presence of networks comprising only of $\alpha1\alpha1\alpha2$(IV)-$\alpha1\alpha1\alpha2$(IV) hexamers. After transplantation, the normal collagen IV, which consists of all the three sets of hexamers, may be recognized as a previously "unseen" antigen with subsequent autoantibody production. However, this autoantibody recognizes a different antigenic epitope and rarely leads to the initiation of overt nephritis [3].

2.4. Clinical presentation

2.4.1. Glomerulonephritis

The commonest disorder is that of the rapidly progressive glomerulonephritis (RPGN). Acute renal injury and oliguria-anuria may evolve within days, whereas slower progression of the renal impairment occurs in a minority of patients. Features of RPGN occur in 80–90% of patients. Macroscopic hematuria may present; however, microscopic hematuria of glomerular origin and red cell casts are the most prominent features. Proteinuria is usually modest. Kidney disease is the only manifestation in 20–40% of patients [16, 17].

2.4.2. *Lung hemorrhage*

Pulmonary and renal involvement occurs in 60–80% of the patients [16]. Cough, dyspnea, hemoptysis, chest pain, hypoxia, iron deficiency and anemia are the presenting manifestations. Pulmonary involvement may precede renal disease by weeks to months [18].

2.4.3. *Systemic manifestations*

Systemic symptoms such as fatigue, arthralgias and fever are infrequent and suggest the coexistence of antineutrophil cytoplasm antibodies (ANCA) vasculitis. Sufficient data regarding the incidence of these symptoms do not exist.

2.5. Renal pathology

Light microscopy reveals diffuse proliferative glomerulonephritis with rupture of the GBM, areas of fibrinoid necrosis and crescent formation in severe disease. Crescents involve approximately 75% of the glomeruli and typically show the same features of activity and chronicity in contrast to other causes of crescentic glomerulonephritis. Tubular injury is proportionate to the degree of crescents. In mild disease, segmental proliferative injury with infiltrating neutrophils and monocytes is observed.

Immunofluorescence demonstrates linear deposition of immunoglobulin G along the GBM. IgA or IgM deposition is rare. Deposition of C3 in a granular pattern is found in approximately 75% of the biopsies. Electron microscopy examination reveals GBM fractures, necrosis and crescents [19].

2.6. Diagnosis

Diagnosis is based on the detection of circulating anti-GBM antibodies in conjunction with the identification of anti-GBM nephritis by kidney biopsy. Anti-GBM antibodies can be detected by indirect immunofluorescence or by direct enzyme-linked immunosorbent assay (ELISA), which has a high sensitivity (95%) and specificity (97%). Positive results are confirmed by Western blot. Indirect immunofluorescence is rarely performed; it has a false-negative rate of 40% and requires an experienced pathologist [20]. ANCA antibodies, mainly with specificity for myeloperoxidase, are found in 10–38% of patients with anti-GBM disease. These patients are characterized as "double positive" [21].

Pulmonary involvement is investigated by chest radiograph and CT scan, broncho-alveolar lavage and pulmonary function testing. Bilateral, patchy consolidations that spare the apices are found on the chest film. A computed tomography (CT) scan reveals widespread areas of ground glass morphology which are not pathognomonic of the disease. Broncho-alveolar lavage shows the characteristic hemosiderin-laden macrophages.

2.7. Therapeutic management

Given the rarity of the disease, the therapeutic management is based on a small number of studies, mainly retrospective ones. The treatment of choice in anti-GBM disease is immunosuppression consisting of corticosteroids and cyclophosphamide in combination with plasma exchange [22].

2.7.1. Immunosuppressive therapy

When the diagnosis is highly suspected, immediate administration of high dose pulse corticosteroids is recommended [22]. Methylprednisolone 500–1000 mg/day for 3 consecutive days, followed by prednisone 1 mg/kg/day orally is the regimen most commonly used. Once the diagnosis is established, oral cyclophosphamide (CYC) at a dose of 2 mg/kg/day must be instituted. Although oral and intravenous CYC have not been compared in this patient population, the latter is used only in unreliable patients or those with severe renal injury to reduce bladder toxicity. Timing of immunosuppression withdrawal is not well established, although maintenance treatment is not recommended [22]. Cyclophosphamide is continued for approximately 3 months and steroids for 6 months. Some experts suggest a shorter duration of therapy (2–3 months) in the case of disease remission and negative antibody titers that persist. In patients with active disease at 3–4 months, immunosuppression comprising steroids and azathioprine may be prolonged up to 6–9 months.

Plasma exchange is generally performed after the diagnosis is confirmed. However, in patients with severe pulmonary hemorrhage, plasmapheresis may begin immediately. Among 17 patients with anti-GBM-induced renal disease, 9 were randomized to prednisone and CYC, whereas 8 also received plasmapheresis. At the end of the therapy, two patients in the plasmapheresis group became dialysis dependent compared to the six patients in the control group [23]. These results were confirmed by a large retrospective study of 221 patients from China [24]. Patient and renal survival rates were better among those who were treated with plasmapheresis in addition to standard immunosuppression. The usual prescription is daily or alternate-day exchanges for 2–3 weeks.

According to the Kidney Disease: Improving Global Outcomes (KDIGO) guidelines, this intense therapeutic regimen applies to all patients with anti-GBM disease. However, dialysis-dependent patients at presentation with approximately 100% crescents on kidney biopsy seem to have a low probability of renal recovery [22, 24]. Therefore, plasma exchange is not advised unless concurrent lung hemorrhage occurs, since the potential complications may exceed the benefits of therapy. Our approach is to perform plasmapheresis regardless of the crescent ratio in:

- Young patients with less comorbidities
- Patients with recent onset of the disease
- Patients with concurrent clinical and laboratory manifestations of ANCA vasculitis

Rituximab has been used as first- or second-line therapy in a limited number of patients with anti-GBM disease, with variable effect on renal function [25, 26].

2.8. Prognosis

In the past, mortality rates of patients with anti-GBM disease due to pulmonary hemorrhage or renal failure were approximately 100%. The combination of aggressive immunosuppression with plasmapheresis has dramatically changed patient survival. Levy et al. have conducted a retrospective study of 71 patients with anti-GBM disease followed for up to 25 years [27]. The therapy consisted of plasmapheresis, high dose oral prednisone and CYC. Serum creatinine (sCr) at presentation seemed to be associated with patient and renal outcome. If the initial sCr was <5.7 mg/dl, the 1-year patient and renal survival rates were 100 and 95%, respectively. At 5 years, the patient and renal survival approached 94%. In the case of severe renal impairment not requiring dialysis at presentation with sCr >5.7 mg/dl, the patient and renal survival rates were 83 and 82%, respectively, at 1 year, and 80 and 50% at 5 years, respectively. Dialysis dependence at presentation correlated to reduced patient survival, 65 and 44% at 1 and 5 years, respectively. Renal recovery was rare in this group and occurred in 8% of the patients at the first year and in 13% of them at 5 years. The proportion of glomerular crescents strongly correlated to the degree of renal impairment. The need for immediate dialysis initiation and 100% crescents on kidney biopsy resulted in irreversible kidney damage despite aggressive treatment.

An interesting study by Yang et al. showed that high levels of anti-GBM antibodies against epitopes EA and EB occur in patients with severe renal damage and correlate to poor prognosis [28].

Patients with positive anti-GBM and ANCA antibodies have a poor renal outcome despite adequate treatment [17]. Relapses are more common in this population, in whom the vasculitis is incriminated [29].

2.9. Renal transplantation

Renal transplantation in patients with anti-GBM disease is delayed until clinical and laboratory quiescence. It is our practice to delay kidney transplantation for at least 6 months after immunosuppression discontinuation. Biopsies of renal allografts show linear deposition of IgG, without symptomatic disease in many patients. Disease recurrence posttransplantation is reported to be 2.7% [30].

De novo anti-GBM disease may develop in 3% of patients with Alport syndrome after renal transplantation [30].

Mutations in the *COL4A5* gene located on the X chromosome are the most frequent as it has already been mentioned, although autosomal recessive and dominant disease have been found. An alloimmune response against the antigens of the kidney allograft leads to the development of anti-GBM antibodies. In this patient group, a second kidney transplantation is associated with a more aggressive disease [31]. Recent guidelines advise the implementation of genetic testing for the evaluation of the risk of de novo disease posttransplantation [32].

2.10. Summary

Anti-GBM disease is an organ-specific autoimmune disorder characterized by the production of autoantibodies against the basement membrane of glomeruli and alveoli. Dominant manifestations are crescentic glomerulonephritis and pulmonary hemorrhage that may be life-threatening. The severity of renal impairment at presentation as well as the need for dialysis and the percent of glomerular crescents are factors prognostic of renal and patient survival. Therefore, early and timely diagnosis is of major importance. Treatment is based on the removal of pathogenetic antibodies by plasma exchange and the prevention of antibody production by a short course of immunosuppressants, namely cyclophosphamide and steroids.

3. Cryoglobulinemic vasculitis

3.1. Introduction

Cryoglobulinemic vasculitis (CV) is a small-vessel vasculitis that affects mainly the skin, the joints, the peripheral nerves and the kidneys. Medium-sized vessels may also be involved. Cryoglobulins are immunoglobulin or immune complexes that precipitate in vitro at temperatures below 37°Cand dissolve upon rewarming [33].

Brouet et al. in 1974 [33] developed a classification system based on the immunoglobulin composition of cryoglobulins:

Type I cryoglobulins are single monoclonal immunoglobulins most often of the IgG or IgM isotype, found in lymphoproliferative disorders, usually Waldenstrom's macroglobulinemia, multiple myeloma and monoclonal gammopathy of unknown significance (MGUS). Type II cryoglobulins are composed of monoclonal IgM with rheumatoid factor (RF) activity in association with polyclonal immunoglobulins (usually IgG). The commonest cause is hepatitis C virus (HCV) infection. Other causes include infection from hepatitis B virus (HBV) or human immunodeficiency virus (HIV), autoimmune diseases and lymphoproliferative disorders. Type III cryoglobulins consist of polyclonal IgM with RF activity and polyclonal IgG. They are linked to autoimmune disorders and infections, mainly due to HCV. Types II and III are associated with mixed cryoglobulinemia (MC) syndrome. In the case of no identifiable cause, type II or III cryoglobulinemia is characterized as essential.

3.2. Epidemiology

The prevalence of CV has been reported to be 1:100,000 individuals [34]. The disease usually occurs between the ages of 45 and 65, with a female predominance (2–3/1). Racial preference has not been recorded. Type I cryoglobulinemia accounts for 10–15% of cryoglobulinemia cases [35]. This type of cryoglobulinemia is most frequently attributed to malignancies of the hematopoietic cells. According to the French nationwide CryoVas survey, among 64 patients with type I CV, 56% suffered from a hematologic malignancy, while MGUS was present in 44% of them [36].

Mixed cryoglobulinemia is reported to be present in approximately 75% of cryoglobulinemias. HCV is the main underlying disorder in 80–90% of individuals with MC [37].

3.3. Pathogenesis of kidney injury in cryoglobulinemic vasculitis

In chronic viral or bacterial infections (hepatitis C, hepatitis B, endocarditis), defective handling of antigenic peptides whether due to high antigenic load or abnormally functioning immune regulatory mechanisms might contribute to a state of persistent antigenemia. The result is the stimulation of an immune response with subsequent release of antigen-directed antibodies and the formation of immune complexes. Impaired antigen clearance due to complement deficiency or to a defect in the reticuloendothelial system may result in the deposition of immune complexes in the glomeruli either by passive trapping of circulating immune complexes or by in situ formation [38]. Monocytes isolated from patients with active cryoglobulinemic glomerulonephritis display delayed processing of cryoglobulins and reduced ability of catabolism, thus favoring tissue deposition [39]. The mesangium and subendothelial space are the sites of immune complex localization.

Subsequent complement activation generates the chemotactic factor C5α which promotes the accumulation of circulating neutrophil and monocytes-macrophages [38]. The association between C5 activation and neutrophil accumulation has been shown in a murine model of cryoglobulin-induced immune complex glomerulonephritis [40]. Moreover, the formation of the terminal membrane attack complex (C5b-9) activates inflammatory cells of the glomerulus to act similarly [40–42]. Leucocytes release acute inflammatory mediators (oxidants, proteases) that damage the capillary wall leading to proteinuria and the decrease of the glomerular filtration rate (GFR). On the other hand, glomerular cells release chemokines and growth factors that mediate direct damage of the glomerulus through matrix accumulation and *mesangial* cell proliferation [6]. The magnitude and severity of glomerular injury seem to be associated to monocyte chemotactic protein-1 (MCP-1) expression [43].

Healthy mice that have been injected with a monoclonal antibody exhibiting both cryoglobulin and rheumatoid factor properties develop cutaneous and glomerular lesions. Moreover, the loss of the rheumatoid factor activity may protect from the development of skin but not glomerular vasculitis, indicating that cryoglobulins alone are sufficient to induce nephritic damage [44].

Pathogenetic mechanisms involved in HCV-associated cryoglobulinemic glomerulonephritis have been more extensively studied. It seems that a nonenveloped core protein, HCV E2, exhibits nephritogenic properties and binds to the complement-fixing antibody IgG3 [45–47]. The complex that is formatted activates the classic complement pathway through C1q and stimulates the production of B-cell clones through binding to B-cell receptors (i.e., CD81 molecule) [47–49]. Monoclonal B lymphocyte expansion seems to be associated to the development of nephritis [50]. Subsequently, monoclonal IgMκ and polyclonal IgG antibodies with rheumatoid factor activity are elicited. Immune complexes consisting of IgG, IgM (identical to those of the cryoprecipitates), viral proteins and complement deposit in the mesangium and subendothelial space causing inflammation and mesangial expansion [46, 49, 51]. It is noteworthy that the autoimmune response may persist even after complete suppression of viremia [52]. Finally, the increased expression of vascular cell adhesion molecule 1 (VCAM-1) has been associated to severe vasculitic lesions in patients with HCV and mixed cryoglobulinemia, a finding that has not been confirmed in patients with kidney involvement. Cryoglobulins act as anti-endothelial antibodies and induce platelet aggregation [45, 53].

3.4. Clinical presentation

3.4.1. Extra-renal manifestations

The "Meltzer's triad" consisting of weakness, purpura and arthralgia is reported in 80% of the patients early in the course of the disease [54]. Palpable purpura of the lower extremities occurs in 70–90% of patients, but Raynaud's phenomenon, acrocyanosis and necrotic ulcers have been described. Arthralgias usually symmetric, involving mainly the large joints, develop in 40–72% of the cases. Sensory or sensory motor polyneuropathy presents with painful paresthesias and motor deficit of the lower limbs in 58–70% of the affected individuals. A minority of the patients may present with mononeuritis multiplex [36, 54–56]. However, hepatic, gastrointestinal, pulmonary, cardiovascular and central nervous system involvement, as well as sicca symptoms, have also been reported [57]. The CryoVas study showed that type I CV seems to be characterized by a higher incidence of severe cutaneous lesions compared to mixed cryoglobulinemia syndrome (50 vs. 30%), whereas severe skin involvement is even more infrequent in HCV-related mixed cryoglobulinemia (5%) [36, 54, 55, 58].

3.4.2. Renal manifestations

Renal damage is present at the time of diagnosis in approximately 20–35% of the patients, whereas 10–35% of them will eventually develop renal disease at some point during the course of the disease [36, 53–55, 59]. Renal manifestations vary. Microscopic hematuria and mild proteinuria occur in nearly 41% of the patients. Nephrotic or nephritic syndrome is less frequent accounting for 22 and 14% of the cases, respectively. The incidence of hypertension is approximately 65%. Other clinical features include acute renal injury or chronic kidney disease [36, 54, 59]. The main pathological pattern, in over 80% of affected individuals, is that of type-I membranoproliferative glomerulonephritis (MPGN) with subendothelial deposits. It seems to be strongly related to type II IgMκ mixed cryoglobulinemia [60].

3.5. Renal pathology

Membranoproliferative glomerulonephritis (MPGN) is the characteristic histopathological pattern observed in mixed cryoglobulinemia. The lesions may be histologically identical to MPGN type I.

Light microscopy reveals varying degrees of glomerular hypercellularity because of the influx of leucocytes. It is often global and diffuse with a predominance of monocytes/macrophages, whereas neutrophils are observed during the acute phase. Monocyte infiltration of the interstitium may also be seen. Mesangial and endocapillary cell proliferation leads to enlargement and lobular accentuation of the glomerular tuft which is typical of the disease. Subendothelial, Periodic acid–Schiff (PAS)-positive eosinophilic deposits are present. Intraluminal thrombi consisting of precipitated cryoglobulins are not a rare finding. However, complete lumen obstruction is uncommon. The severity of clinical manifestations seems to be related to the extent of endocapillary proliferation and the abundance of glomerular deposits. Mesangial matrix expansion and accumulation and the interposition of mesangial cells, monocytes and endothelial cells lead to the appearance of double-contoured glomerular basement membrane (GBM) which is recognized by PAS and silver staining. Extracapillary proliferation is a rare finding. Vasculitic lesions of small- and middle-sized renal arteries are described in approximately 30% of the cases. They comprise vascular PAS-positive deposits, endoluminal accumulation of leucocytes and fibrinoid necrotizing vasculitis in more advanced stages of the disease.

Direct immunofluorescence examination shows granular glomerular and luminal deposits that stain positive for both IgM and IgG in type II, III cryoglobulinemia. Subendothelial and mesangial deposits may also contain C3 and less frequently components of the classical complement pathway (C1q, C4).

Electron microscopy reveals the deposits that can be either amorphous or organized into curved and annular fibrils with a tubular appearance in cross-section and a diameter of 20–35 nm [60, 61].

3.6. Diagnosis and laboratory findings

Criteria for the classification of CV have been proposed [62]. Three parameters (questionnaire, clinical, laboratory findings) have been taken into account.

1. Patients are classified as having CV, if at least two of the three items are positive.
2. The patient must be positive for serum cryoglobulins in at least two determinations at 12 weeks' interval or less.
3. Questionnaire item: at least two out of the following: (1) Do you remember one or more episodes of small red spots on your skin, particularly involving the lower limbs? (2) Have you ever had red spots on your lower extremities, which leave a brownish color after their disappearance? (3) Has a doctor ever told you that you have viral hepatitis?
4. Clinical item: at least three out of the following four (present or past) (1) Constitutional symptoms: fatigue, low-grade fever, or fever >388C of no other cause, fibromyalgia. (2) Articular involvement, namely arthralgias, arthritis. (3) Vascular involvement: purpura, skin ulcers, necrotizing vasculitis, hyperviscosity syndrome, Raynaud's phenomenon. (4) Neurologic involvement of the peripheral or central nervous system.
5. Laboratory item: at least two out of the following three (present) (1) Low serum C4. (2) Positive serum rheumatoid factor. (3) Serum M component present.

The diagnosis of CV with kidney involvement is based on clinical manifestations in the presence of cryoglobulinemia and biopsy-proven MPGN type I.

In type I cryoglobulinemia, precipitation at 1–4°C occurs within hours, whereas in the mixed types precipitation may be delayed. Therefore, samples should be stored for 7 days. When the test is negative in the context of high suspicion, it should be repeated after assuring the correct technique for sampling and handling of the blood. In the case of cryoglobulinemia, the cryocrit, which is the centrifuged volume of the precipitate as a percentage of the original serum volume should be measured if possible. Cryoglobulin concentration > 20–50 mcg/ml or a cryocrit >0.5–1% is considered positive. Cryocrit levels do not correlate with response to the treatment. Furthermore, electrophoresis and immunofixation are performed to determine the exact type of cryoglobulins.

Other surrogate markers indicative of this disorder are RF, acute phase reactants (erythrocyte sedimentation rate and C-reactive protein) and complement components (C1q, C4, CH50). Serological studies for viral infections, urinalysis with examination of the sediment, assessment of renal function and proteinuria should always be included in the evaluation of patients with mixed cryoglobulinemia.

3.7. Prognosis

Cryoglobulinemic vasculitis is associated with significant morbidity and mortality. In HCV-related mixed CV, 1-year and 10-year survival rate is estimated to be 96 and 63%, respectively. Factors prognostic of a poor outcome are severe liver fibrosis, central nervous system and kidney and/or cardiac involvement [58]. In noninfectious mixed CV, age > 65 years, pulmonary and gastrointestinal involvement and renal impairment with GFR < 60 ml/min seem to be independently linked to death [56]. Main causes of death are infections and cardiovascular disease [56, 58]. In type I CV, 1- and 10-year survival rate is higher, 97 and 87%, respectively [36].

3.8. Therapeutic management

The therapeutic management of glomerulonephritis in CV depends on the underlying etiological disorder and the severity of the disease.

3.8.1. Therapeutic management of mixed cryoglobulinemic vasculitis

The therapeutic regimen comprises immunosuppression in selected cases as well as treatment of the underlying disorder.

3.8.1.1. Immunosuppressive therapy

The main indication for immunosuppressive therapy in patients with renal involvement is glomerulonephritis associated with a rapidly progressive pattern and/or nephrotic syndrome. In the case of severe, organ-threatening disease, immunosuppression is instituted immediately, even prior to disease-specific therapy. This does not apply to patients with HIV or HBV infection who should always receive effective antiviral treatment in order to eradicate viremia before immunosuppression use.

Immunosuppression consists of Rituximab and/or corticosteroids. Data supporting the use of cyclophosphamide are limited, whereas plasmapheresis should also be considered in severe disease [63].

3.8.1.2. Rituximab

Cryoglobulinemic vasculitis, especially in the case of HCV infection, is characterized by clonal B-cell expansion, production of IgM and IgG antibodies and immune complex deposition. Rituximab is a chimeric IgG1κ monoclonal antibody targeted against CD20, which is an antigen expressed on the B-cell surface from the early pre-B-cell stage to the activated mature cell stage. The rationale behind the use of rituximab in this patient population is that B-cell depletion may decrease the production of pathogenic cryoglobulins. Moreover, there is evidence that rituximab therapy is not associated with HCV replication, although there are data of HCV viremia without clinical manifestations after Rituximab infusion [64, 65].

In a single-center randomized controlled trial (RCT) [64], 24 patients with HCV-associated mixed cryoglobulinemia were randomized either to receive rituximab (375 mg/m^2/week for 4 weeks) or to continue their current immunosuppressive medications (control group). Antivirals had failed to induce clinical remission in all the patients. At the study entry, 33% of the patients had active glomerulonephritis (four patients in each group). After 6 months, remission defined by a Birmingham Vasculitis Activity Score of zero, was achieved in significantly more patients in the rituximab group (83 vs. 8.3%, $p < 0.001$). Remission sustained for a median of 7 months. In addition, during the 6-month period, patients with nephritis in the control group experienced a decline in renal function whereas rituximab-treated patients had a stable or improved estimated glomerular filtration rate (GFR). However, only three patients in the control group received immunosuppressants, namely low dose corticosteroids (mean dose of 10 mg prednisone daily). On the other hand, of the 12 patients in the intervention group, 6 also received glucocorticoids (mean dose of 26 mg prednisone daily), 1 received cyclophosphamide and 2 were also treated with plasmapheresis. Clinical or laboratory findings indicative of hepatitis were not recorded in either group.

De Vita et al. [66] evaluated the use of Rituximab in 59 patients with CV and severe manifestations (skin ulcers, active glomerulonephritis or peripheral neuropathy). The majority of the patients (93%) had HCV-associated disease, but antiviral therapy failed to achieve remission or was contraindicated. Enrolled patients were randomized either to rituximab therapy (1000 mg at baseline and at day 14) or to conventional treatments (either glucocorticoids, azathioprine or cyclophosphamide, or plasmapheresis). At 12 months, success of the initial treatment was achieved in significantly more patients in the rituximab arm (64.3 vs. 3.5%, $p < 0.0001$). Among seven patients with glomerulonephritis treated with rituximab, complete or partial response was recorded in four of them after 6 months of therapy. Of eight patients with renal involvement under conventional therapy who had a treatment failure, six had a favorable response to rituximab.

The abovementioned studies indicate that rituximab may be a safe and effective treatment in patients with mixed cryoglobulinemia and severe manifestations, especially when HCV antiviral therapy fails to induce remission.

Data regarding the use of rituximab in non-HCV infectious cryoglobulinemia syndrome are scarce. Prompt initiation of antiviral therapy is mandatory in the case of HBV- or HIV-infected patients, since rituximab has been associated with virus reactivation in untreated patient populations [67, 68]. In our opinion, this monoclonal antibody should not be used in patients with HIV infection who are not receiving antiretroic agents and/or have not achieved a virological response. In the case of HBV infection, rituximab should be administered in patients with suppressed viremia under appropriate antiviral therapy. In these patients, the use of immunosuppression alone is associated with a poor response to therapy, whereas remission was reached with antiviral medications. Especially in refractory disease, the combination of antiinfectious agents with immunosuppressants leads to a favorable response [69].

Finally, limited data exist regarding the use of Rituximab in noninfectious CV. The CryoVas survey analyzed data of 242 patients with mixed CV [55]. Causative disorders were connective tissue diseases, essential disease and hematologic malignancies. The therapeutic management was evaluated in 209 patients. Corticosteroid monotherapy or steroids in conjunction with an alkylating agent resulted in lower response rates compared to rituximab with corticosteroids. First-line treatment with rituximab and glucocorticoids allowed for reductions in steroid dosing and was more efficacious in achieving complete renal and clinical response. However, this combination was related to a ninefold higher rate of infections compared to the other regimens. Therefore, although rituximab seems to be a valuable and effective treatment for noninfectious CV, cautiousness regarding the incidence of infections is warranted.

3.8.1.3. Corticosteroids

The use of corticosteroids for the treatment of HCV-associated CV is controversial as there are no randomized controlled trials evaluating their safety and efficacy in this disease. In patients with severe renal involvement, we and other centers administer a short course of high-dose pulse corticosteroids (500–750 mg for 3 consecutive days) followed by oral prednisone 1 mg/kg/day for 2–4 weeks and a rapid tapering to a maintenance dose of 5–10 mg/day, depending on the clinical response. The abovementioned randomized controlled studies [64, 67] included different steroid regimens applied by different investigators in all patients with severe disease and renal injury. Therefore, we cannot conclude regarding potential benefits and the safety profile.

In a small cohort study, five patients with HCV-related cryoglobulinemic glomerulonephritis received rituximab without steroids. Although they all experienced remission of the disease, relapse occurred in four of them from month 5 to month 12 of follow-up [70].

Given the lack of convincing evidence regarding the use of steroids in mixed CV, we believe that high-dose corticosteroids should be used in the management of renal disease. Rapid tapering and concomitant administration of antiinfectious agents are of major importance, since steroid use carries the risk of enhancing viral reactivation.

3.8.1.4. Cyclophosphamide

The benefits and risks of cyclophosphamide (CYC) use in patients with mixed CV cannot be evaluated from the current literature. Cyclophosphamide is not routinely used in patients with HCV cryoglobulinemic vasculitis, since it may increase viral replication or aggravate liver injury. In clinical practice, it may be considered when rituximab therapy fails or when it is unavailable or poorly tolerated. According to the European League Against Rheumatism (EULAR), noninfectious CV can be treated with immunosuppressants including cyclophosphamide [71]. When used, CYC is combined with plasma exchange and it is administered orally at a dose of 2 mg/kg/day for 3 months [67].

3.8.1.5. Plasma exchange

Case reports or small case series have shown that after plasma exchange response occurs in 70–80% of patients with mixed CV. It is performed in cases of organ and/or life-threatening diseases [72], such as:

- Symptomatic hyperviscosity syndrome
- Rapidly progressive glomerulonephritis, MPGN with renal impairment
- Alveolar hemorrhage or acute gastrointestinal vasculitis

It is advised to warm the albumin solution, since acute kidney injury due to cryoglobulin precipitation has been reported [72].

Plasma exchange is always used in combination with immunosuppressive therapy in order to remove circulating cryoglobulins but also to prevent further formation.

3.8.1.6. Treatment of the underlying disorder

3.8.1.6.1. Treatment of hepatitis C or hepatitis B infection

During the past decades, patients with HCV-related cryoglobulinemic vasculitis have been treated with interferon-containing regimens. The introduction of direct acting antiviral agents (DAAs) has radically changed the treatment of patients with HCV infection. These drugs target nonstructural (NS) viral proteins and inhibit HCV replication [73]. Although the efficacy of DAAs in HCV-associated cryoglobulinemic vasculitis has not been confirmed, they are more potent regimens with a better safety profile and a shorter duration of therapy. Taking into account that DAAs are first-line agents in HCV treatment according to current guidelines [74], we believe that they should be offered to patients with CV and hepatitis C. In a prospective study, Gragnani et al. [75] evaluated the efficacy, safety and virological response of different combinations of DAAs in 44 patients with HCV-related cryoglobulinemic vasculitis. Concurrent immunosuppression was given to two patients. Kidney involvement was recorded in four cases. Sustained virologic response and complete clinical remission was achieved in all patients at week 24. Renal function as well as proteinuria ameliorated substantially in patients with renal disease. Adverse events were mild and did not lead to drug discontinuation.

The optimal timing for initiation of antivirals is not clear. It has been recommended to delay antiviral therapy for 1–4 months [63, 71]. The purpose of this approach is to avoid immune-mediated events attributed to interferon regimens. On the other hand, immunosuppression may improve renal function, enhancing the use of DAAs. The proper timing of DAAs' introduction needs to be determined.

Patients with hepatitis B-associated CV and nephritis are treated with entecavir which is associated with less nephrotoxicity and lower rates of resistance. Antiviral therapy not only prevents from HBV replication but it may also induce disease remission [76]. Ideally, it should precede immunosuppressive therapy, which is not recommended in active hepatitis.

3.8.2. Therapeutic management of type I cryoglobulinemic vasculitis

The treatment of type I CV is that of the causative hematological disorder. Rituximab, bortezomib, CYC, lenalidomide and thalidomide have been used with satisfactory results.

More specifically, a bortezomib-based regimen is used in patients with deteriorated renal function, whereas lenalidomide is preferred in cases of neurologic involvement [77]. Rituximab infusion, which has been hypothesized to induce B-cell apoptosis and cryoglobulin release in these patients, seems to be associated with a rapid disease flare [34]. Therefore, rituximab is suggested for use after inducing an initial remission with other treatment regimens [78].

3.9. Summary

- Cryoglobulinemic vasculitis is a small-vessel vasculitis which mainly affects the skin, the joints, the peripheral nerves and the kidneys.
- Etiological factors include chronic viral infections particularly HCV, autoimmune disorders and B-cell lymphoproliferative disorders.
- Renal involvement may be manifested as mild proteinuria with microscopic hematuria, nephrotic or nephritic syndrome and varying degrees of renal impairment. Hypertension is common.
- The predominant histological pattern is MPGN type I. Recent studies have identified prognostic factors that need to be evaluated in clinical trials.
- Treatment strategy is individualized according to the underlying disorder and the severity of the disease. The therapeutic regimen comprises immunosuppression mainly Rituximab in selected cases as well as the treatment of the underlying disorder.

4. IgA vasculitis (Henoch-Schonlein purpura)

4.1. Historical background

IgA vasculitis (IgAV), until recently known as "Henoch-Schonlein purpura," has actually first been described by Heberden in 1806. Later on, in 1837, Schoenlein first described the association of purpuric rash with arthritis, and his student, Henoch, in 1874, added the renal and gastrointestinal involvement to the entity [79–81].

4.2. Nomenclature/organ involvement

According to the 2012 Revised International Chapel Hill Consensus Conference Nomenclature of Vasculitides, the term "Henoch-Schoenlein Purpura" was replaced by "IgA vasculitis" on the basis of the pathophysiological mechanism which is characterized by circulation and tissue deposition of abnormal IgA [1].

According to the new classification, IgAV is an immune complex small-vessel vasculitis (SVV). IgAV may present as a single-organ disease, for example, as isolated cutaneous vasculitis or as renal-limited IgAV which is indistinguishable from IgA nephropathy (IgAN), or as a systemic disease with multiorgan involvement. Patients with initial single-organ involvement may subsequently develop systemic manifestations.

The "classic triad" of organ involvement in IgAV comprises skin involvement manifested as palpable purpura mostly of the lower extremities, arthralgia or arthritis and gastrointestinal manifestations including abdominal pain and occult or overt GI bleeding. Though not included in the classic triad, renal involvement is frequent, occurring in 45–50% of adult patients with IgAV, and is the most important determinant of outcome [82].

4.3. Epidemiology

IgAV is the most common vasculitis in childhood with an annual incidence of 13–20 cases per 100,000 children, affecting most commonly children in the age group of 4–7 years, with a predominance in boys. In children, there is a peak incidence in autumn and winter and the clinical presentation is often preceded by a respiratory infection, suggesting a possible implication of viruses and bacteria as a trigger for the disease [83].

Of these pathogens, the most studied is group-A β hemolytic streptococcus, found in 20–50% of children with IgAV, either as positive throat cultures or by serology as elevated antistreptolysin titers [84].

In adults, IgAV occurs far less frequently and has an annual incidence of 0.8–1.8 per 10,000. There is no seasonal variation in incidence. There is a male predominance with a male to female ratio of 5:1 [82].

IgAV is described worldwide and in all ethnic groups, but its annual incidence, as examined in a worldwide study by Garner-Medwin et al. including children of all origins, has been reported to be lower in the Black race. The ethnic variation of its renal limited counterpart, IgAN, with increased frequency in Japan and East-Asia, less prevalence in Europe and Australia and the lowest prevalence in Africa, has not been detected in IgAV [83, 85, 86].

4.4. Pathophysiology

In recent years, an association between adulthood IgAV and malignancy, as with other autoimmune diseases, has been reported. In a retrospective study including 200 patients with ANCA-associated vasculitis (AASV) and 129 patients with IgAV, the relative risk of malignancy was increased at 6.02 in AASV and 5.25 in IgAV patients, respectively, compared to an age-matched control group of the general population [87].

In the largest cohort of adult patients with IgAV with long-term follow-up, Pillebout et al. report a mortality rate of 26% at 15 years. Malignancy was the leading cause of death in 30% of patients. Almost all of them were solid tumors, most of them being lung and GI carcinomas [88].

Besides solid tumors, IgAV has also been described in the setting of hematologic malignancies as lymphoma and IgA myeloma but also as secondary to infections, vaccines and medications [89–92].

Though there is no proven causal relationship, it seems that, irrespective of the trigger, extrinsic factors, in the presence of a specific genetic background, lead to initiation of the pathogenetic mechanism in IgAV [93].

As for IgAN, the key pathogenetic mechanism includes aberrant glycosylation of the IgA1 isotype of IgA. According to the "multihit hypothesis," this galactose-deficient IgA1 induces autoantibody production toward the neoantigen. These antiglycan antibodies bind to the abnormal IgA1 leading to complement activation via the alternate or the lectin pathway and to the subsequent formation of immune complexes, which deposit in the affected organs [94].

4.5. Differential diagnosis and diagnostic criteria

The typical presentation of IgAV includes palpable purpuric rash of the lower extremities, gastro-intestinal bleeding and/or abdominal pain, arthralgia or arthritis and in case of renal involvement, microscopic hematuria and subnephrotic proteinuria with or without renal function impairment.

In cases of more atypical presentation, especially in adulthood, other diseases with similar clinical features must be excluded. Immune thrombocytopenic purpura (ITP) and thrombotic microangiopathies may present with a hemorrhagic rash but can easily be excluded by the absence of thrombocytopenia or hemolysis [95].

Cryoglobulinemic, urticarial and hypersensitivity vasculitides may also present with skin lesions, arthritis and renal involvement. In this setting, a skin biopsy, when performed adequately involving active lesions, may confirm the diagnosis of IgAV. The typical histologic features are those of leukocytoclastic vasculitis with fibrinoid necrosis and perivascular infiltration of leukocytes and monocytes. On immunofluorescence, there is IgA deposition along with C3 and fibrin [96].

In the minority of cases with predominance of GI symptoms that may precede the other manifestations, causes of surgical abdomen must be ruled out.

There are no distinctive laboratory parameters for the diagnosis of IgAV. Serum levels of IgA may be increased in about 50% of patients and rarely complement components C3, and C4 might be decreased [97].

A series of diagnostic criteria including clinical and laboratory parameters and histologic features of skin biopsy for the diagnosis of IgAV have been proposed. The first attempt was in 1990 by the American College of Rheumatology (ACR) which were revised and extended first by Michel in 1992, later on by Helander, de Castro and Gibson in 1995, coming to the more recent EULAR/PRINTO/PRESS Criteria in 2010. The extended description and comparison of the sensitivity and specificity of these criteria have been published by Yang et al. in 2014. Most data for the diagnostic criteria have been derived from studies in pediatric populations [98].

4.6. Clinical manifestations

4.6.1. Purpura

The typical presentation is palpable purpura, often symmetric, predominantly affecting the lower extremities, at pressure sites, but it can extend to the whole body. In children, rash most often resolves spontaneously after 2–3 weeks and may relapse in about one-third of patients. In adults, in about 30% of patients, it may present with more severe forms including blisters, hemorrhagic and necrotic lesions [99].

4.6.2. Joint involvement

The second most common manifestation affecting about 75% of patients is joint pain, most often of the knees and ankles, impairing walking. Overt arthritis is less common [97].

4.6.3. Gastrointestinal involvement

GI involvement occurs in about 50–75% of patients with IgAV. The presenting symptom is most often colicky abdominal pain which occurs typically soon, in about 2–10 days after the onset of rash. In a minority of patients (10–20%), abdominal symptoms may precede the onset of purpura; in this setting diagnosis may be difficult. Occult GI bleeding is common in IgAV, while gross bleeding with melanotic or hemorrhagic stools occurs in less than 10% of patients. The most frequently involved sites of the GI tract are the duodenum and the small intestine. Esophagogastroduodenoscopy (EGD) is the preferred diagnostic procedure in patients with suspected IgAV. The typical findings are irregular ulcers and petechiae in the duodenum. Small intestine radiography and colonoscopy may also be necessary. Severe GI complications as intussusception and perforation occur in 1–5% of patients [100].

4.6.4. Renal involvement

Renal involvement occurs in about 25–54% of children and in 45–85% of adults with IgAV. In adults, it is a rare entity, which accounts for 0.6–2% of all biopsy-proven glomerulonephritides. In adults, there is not only increased frequency of renal involvement but also a worse outcome compared to children. Reported progression rates to ESRD in children range from 5 to 10%, while in adults they reach 30% and more [101].

4.6.5. Clinical presentation

The most common clinical manifestation is microscopic hematuria with subnephrotic proteinuria in 80% of patients. In contrast to IgAN, macroscopic hematuria is less common in IgAV. Arterial hypertension and impaired renal function are present in about 30% of adults at disease onset. About 10–20% of adult patients present with nephritic or nephrotic syndrome [82].

Renal biopsy is performed more often in adults than in children, in whom the disease is generally mild and resolves spontaneously. In adulthood, the necessity of a renal biopsy is implicated by the rarity of the disease, the differential diagnosis between other small-vessel vasculitides as AASV or cryoglobulinemic vasculitis or in the setting of rapid deterioration of renal function or severe renal impairment at presentation.

4.7. Histology

Histological lesions of IgAV are indistinguishable from IgAN with the diagnostic hallmark being prominent IgA deposition in the mesangium by immunofluorescence staining. Concurrent deposition of C3 and less commonly IgG and IgM may also be present. On light microscopy, the most common finding is mesangial hypercellularity and mesangial matrix expansion. Electron microscopy examination reveals electron-dense material corresponding to the immune-complex deposition, predominantly in the mesangium. Histologic features in patients with IgAV as with IgAN have enormous variations in terms of activity and chronicity, the former including endocapillary proliferation, fibrinoid necrosis and cellular crescents and the latter comprising focal and/or segmental glomerulosclerosis, adhesions to Bowman's capsule, interstitial fibrosis and tubular atrophy, respectively [102].

In IgAN, according to the Oxford Classification, the histologic features were found to be prognostic indicators of renal outcome long term: mesangial hypercellularity, endocapillary proliferation, segmental glomerulosclerosis or adhesion and tubular atrophy and interstitial fibrosis (MEST score) [103].

In a retrospective cohort of 250 adult patients with IgAV, Pillebout et al. analyzed renal involvement and renal outcome parameters. In this study, a different classification scheme in order to determine histologic features as prognostic indicators was introduced for IgAV. This classification divides IgAV into five classes based on the severity of active as endo- and extra-capillary proliferation (classes 3a and 3b) and chronic lesions as fibrotic kidney with global sclerosis in more than 50% of glomeruli (class V), respectively [88].

This histological approach is preferable compared to the Oxford Classification adopted from IgAN, since patients with IgAV have worse initial presentation and possibly outcome compared to IgAN, while in the Oxford study, patients with severe renal impairment (eGFR <30 ml/min) and rapidly progressive glomerulonephritis (RPGN) were excluded [103].

4.8. Outcome

The most relevant studies are summarized in **Table 1**. Almost all studies are retrospective and include children and adults.

A *multicenter* observational study from Italy included 95 adults and 57 children with a mean follow-up of 5 years. The authors report similar outcomes in terms of remission rates (32.5% in adults vs. 31.5% in children) and survival rates at 5 years (85 and 95%, respectively) [104]. On the other hand, a retrospective study from Spain including 116 children and 46 adults with IgAV nephritis, with a relatively short-term follow-up of 15 months, reported more frequent and severe renal involvement in adults, with high complete recovery rates at 89% in the adult and 94% in the children group, respectively [105].

Among adults, the reported rates of ESRD range from 8–16% at 5–15 years [88, 104, 106]. Proteinuria >1 g/day [88, 104, 106], impaired renal function at presentation [88, 104] and arterial hypertension [104] have been identified as negative prognostic indicators.

4.9. Therapy of renal manifestations

Currently, most of the evidence for the therapy of IgAV nephritis comes from retrospective cohorts including children and adults. According to the KDIGO Guidelines of 2012, "IgAV nephritis in adults should be treated the same as in children" (weak evidence, level of recommendation 2D) [22].

Study	Number of patients	Follow-up (years)	CKD	ESRD	Death	Recovery	Prognostic indicators
Retrospective Multicenter Italy; Coppo et al. [104]	95 adults 57 children	5	This endpoint was not included in the study	16% 7%	This endpoint was not included in the study	32% 31%	↓GFR; Proteinuria >1 g/day; Arterial hypertension
Retrospective Spain; Blanco et al. [105]	116 children 46 adults	1.8	This endpoint was not included in the study	This endpoint was not included in the study	This endpoint was not included in the study	94% 89%	This endpoint was not included in the study
Retrospective Finland; Rauta et al. [106]	38 adults	6	19%	8%	This endpoint was not included in the study	This endpoint was not included in the study	Proteinuria >1 g/day
Retrospective Multicenter France; Pillebout et al. [88]	250 adults	15	38%	11%	26%	This endpoint was not included in the study	Proteinuria >1 g/day; Initial GFR < 50 ml/min

Table 1. Outcome of patients with IgA vasculitis.

On the other hand, almost all studies have shown more frequent and more severe renal involvement in adult IgAV nephritis with worse prognosis and outcome; therefore, it is indeed a weak suggestion to treat a disease with a different clinical picture and outcome the same as in a dissimilar patient population as children, who often have an indolent self-limiting nephritis course [88, 104–106].

The only RCT investigating treatment of IgAV nephritis in adults was a 12-month, prospective, open-label trial, the CESAR study. This study included 54 adult patients with severe, proliferative IgAV nephritis excluding those with RPGN. Patients were randomized to receive either steroid monotherapy or steroids with cyclophosphamide. The study showed that there was no additional benefit in renal outcome in the steroid and cyclophosphamide group. However, one must consider that the study was underpowered, since the number of patients was relatively low and follow-up time short [107].

With regard to the KDIGO Guidelines for the therapy of IgAV nephritis [22], as mentioned earlier, the suggestion is to treat the disease the same as in children while recommendations in children refer to the recommendations for IgAN. Taking into consideration that it is difficult to perform RCTs in adults in a rare entity as IgAV and that it is even more difficult to extrapolate data from children into adults, the most reasonable approach is to treat renal involvement in adult IgAV based on the recommendations for adult IgAN.

Since IgAN is probably the glomerulonephritis with the broader spectrum of clinical presentations and histologic features of active and chronic lesions, therapeutic benefit must outweigh long-term toxicity, especially in a disease with chronic course and often irreversible damage at presentation.

A very pragmatic approach for the treatment of IgAN, that can be applied to IgAV nephritis, since histological features and central pathogenetic mechanisms are identical, has been published by Floege and Eitner in 2011 [108].

IgAN patients can be divided into four clinical categories and therapeutic interventions must be tailored based on these entities. Mild renal involvement.

The first patient group the so-called "silent majority" involves all patients in whom the disease is diagnosed incidentally, who present with isolated microscopic hematuria and who in fact even do not fulfill strict criteria for performing a renal biopsy. Those patients only need long-term follow-up for up to 10 years, which is indeed difficult to achieve in otherwise healthy individuals.

Moderate renal involvement.

The second category comprises the "typical IgAN patient" with micro- and macroscopic hematuria, subnephrotic proteinuria, presence or absence of arterial hypertension and preserved renal function at diagnosis. These patients should be treated with general supportive measures and if proteinuria persists above 1 g/day, they should receive a 6-month course of high-dose steroid monotherapy. This approach has shown benefit in terms of preserving renal function while mycophenolate acid has not proven efficacy, at least in Caucasian populations, and combination of steroids with other immunosuppressive agents has not shown additional benefits. In the stop-IgAN trial, addition of immunosuppression to optimized supportive treatment in patients of this category did not show a beneficial effect after a follow-up of 3 years [109].

4.9.1. Severe renal involvement

4.9.1.1. Severely impaired renal function

The third category is those patients with severely impaired renal function. The "point of no return" is defined as a creatinine level above 2.5–3.0 mg/dl or an eGFR <30 ml/min. In this patient group, optimizing supportive treatment is mandatory while immunosuppression has no indication and may be even harmful.

4.9.1.2. Rapid deterioration of renal function or nephrotic syndrome

The fourth group includes rare manifestations as rapid deterioration of renal function or nephrotic syndrome. In the case of *rapidly increased creatinine*, a repeat biopsy should be performed within 5–10 days in order to differentiate between RPGN and acute tubular injury (ATI) due to tubular obliteration by red cell casts [110].

In the case of RPGN, according to KDIGO Guidelines, treatment with steroids and cyclophosphamide as for ANCA-associated vasculitis is suggested (level 2D of recommendation) [111, 112].

In the rare cases of overt nephrotic syndrome, therapy as for minimal change disease (MCD) is indicated [113].

4.10. Therapy of systemic manifestations

Corticosteroids are ineffective in shortening the course or the severity of skin lesions as well as in preventing relapses of purpura. The alkaloid drug colchicine at low doses of 1 mg/day, the antibacterial drug Dapsone and the leukotriene receptor antagonist Montelukast have been used in a small series of patients including predominantly children, with satisfactory results but with limited efficacy in terms of preventing relapses [114–116].

For gastrointestinal and joint involvement, steroids are effective and are considered first-line treatment as monotherapy [117].

4.11. Summary

- IgAV in adults represents a rare entity which should always be included in the differential diagnosis of a patient presenting with nephritic features and skin rash.
- The disease differs from that in children; in adults, it has been associated with solid tumors whereas in children it is often triggered by viral or bacterial infections. In adults there is no seasonal clustering and the male predominance exists, but to a lesser degree. Most importantly, children have a more indolent, self-limiting disease course, while in adults, clinical presentation and outcomes are worse.
- Renal involvement is more frequent in adults with more severe manifestations and worse disease course which progresses to CKD/ESRD in about 30% of patients. Similarly, to IgAN and other glomerulonephritides, indicators of poor prognosis include persistent proteinuria, impaired renal function and hypertension at diagnosis. The central pathogenetic mechanism and the renal histologic features are identical to IgAN, strongly suggesting that IgAN may represent a single-organ variant of systemic IgAV. Therapeutic recommendations for IgAV are extrapolated from studies in children and, more correctly, from IgAN.
- Though our understanding of IgAV has improved over the last few years, several questions about the pathogenetic mechanisms, the genetic predisposition, the determinants of outcome and the optimal therapeutic approach still remain unanswered.

Author details

Smaragdi Marinaki, Chrysanthi Skalioti, Sophia Lionaki and John N. Boletis*

*Address all correspondence to: laikneph@laiko.gr

Faculty of Medicine, Laiko Hospital, National and Kapodistrian University of Athens, Greece

References

[1] Jennete JC. Overview of the 2012 revised international Chapel Hill Concensus conference nomenclature of Vasculitides. Clinical and Experimental Nephrology. 2013;**17**(5):603-606. DOI: 10.1007/s10157-013-0869-6

[2] Goodpasture EW. The significance of certain pulmonary lesions in relation to the etiology of pneumonia. The American Journal of the Medical Sciences. 1919;**158**:863-870

[3] Krakower CA, Greenspon SA. Localization of the nephrotoxic antigen within the isolated renal glomerulus. A.M.A. Archives of Pathology. 1951;**51**:629-639

[4] Lerner RA, Glassock RJ, Dixon FJ. The role of anti-glomerular basement membrane antibody in the pathogenesis of human glomerulonephritis. The Journal of Experimental Medicine. 1967;**126**:989-1004

[5] Fomegné G, Dratwa M, Wens R, et al. Goodpasture disease. Revue Médicale de Bruxelles. 2006;**27**:162-166. [Article in French]

[6] Peto P, Salama AD. Update on antiglomerular basement membrane disease. Current Opinion in Rheumatology. 2011;**23**:32-37. DOI: 10.1097/BOR.0b013e328341009f

[7] Cui Z, Zhao MH. Advances in human antiglomerular basement membrane disease. Nature Reviews. Nephrology. 2011;**7**:697-705. DOI: 10.1038/nrneph.2011.89

[8] Sundaramoorthy M, Meiyappan M, Todd P, Hudson BG. Crystal structure of NC1 domains: Structural basis for type IV collagen assembly in basement membranes. The Journal of Biological Chemistry. 2002;**277**:31142-31153. DOI: 10.1074/jbc.M201740200

[9] Harvey SJ, Zheng K, Sado Y, et al. Role of distinct type IV collagen networks in glomerular development and function. Kidney International. 1998;**54**:1857-1866

[10] Hudson BG, Tryggvason, Sundaramoorthy M, Neilson EG. Alport's syndrome, Goodpasture's syndrome and type IV collagen. NEngl. Journal of Medicine. 2003;**348**:2543-2556

[11] Pedchenko V, Bondar O, Fogo AB, et al. Molecular architecture of the Goodpastureautoantigen in anti-GBM nephritis. The New England Journal of Medicine. 2010;**363**:343. DOI: 10.1056/nejmoa0910500

[12] Rutgers A, Meyers KE, Canziani G, et al. High affinity of anti-GBM antibodies from Goodpasture and transplanted Alport patients to alpha3(IV)NC1 collagen. Kidney International. 2000;**58**:115

[13] Cui Z, Wang HY, Zhao MH. Natural autoantibodies against glomerular basement membrane exist in normal human sera. Kidney International. 2006;**69**:894. DOI: 10.1038/sj.ki.5000135

[14] Wu J, Hicks J, Borillo J, Glass WF II, Lou YH. CD4(+) T cells specific to a glomerular basement membrane antigen mediate glomerulonephritis. The Journal of Clinical Investigation. 2002;**109**:517-524. DOI: 10.1172/JCI13876

[15] Phelps RG, Rees AJ. The HLA complex in Goodpasture's disease: A model for analyzing susceptibility to autoimmunity. Kidney International. 1999;**56**:1638-1653

[16] Hellmark T, Segelmark M. Diagnosis and classification of Goodpasture's disease (anti-GBM). Journal of Autoimmunity. 2014;**48-49**:108-112. DOI: 10.1016/j.jaut.2014.01.024

[17] Srivastava A, Rao GK, Segal PE, Shah M, Geetha D. Characteristics and outcome of crescentic glomerulonephritis in patients with both antineutrophil cytoplasmic antibody and anti-glomerular basement membrane antibody. Clinical Rheumatology. 2013;**32**:1317-1312. DOI: 10.1007/s10067-013-2268-5

[18] Lazor R, Bigay-Game L, Cottin V, Cadranel J, Decaux O, Fellrath JM, et al. Alveolar hemorrhage in anti-basement membrane antibody disease: A series of 28 cases. Medicine (Baltimore). 2007;**86**:181e93. DOI: 10.1097/md

[19] Fogo AB, Lusso MA, Najafian B, Alpers CE. AJKD atlas of renal pathology: Anti–glomerular basement membrane antibody–mediated glomerulonephritis. Atlas of renal pathology II. Fogo AB editor. American Journal of Kidney Diseases. 2016;**68**(5):e29-e30. DOI: 10.1053/S0272-6386(13)90008-1

[20] Sinico RA, Radice A, Corace C, Sabadini E, Bollini B. Anti-glomerular basement membrane antibodies in the diagnosis of Goodpasture syndrome: A comparison of different assays. Nephrology, Dialysis, Transplantation. 2006;**21**:397-401

[21] Levy JB, Hammad T, Coulthart A, Dougan T, Pusey CD. Clinical features and outcome of patients with both ANCA and anti-GBM antibodies. Kidney International. 2004;**66**(4):1535-1540

[22] Kidney Disease. Improving global outcomes (KDIGO) glomerulonephritis work group. KDIGO clinical practice guideline for glomerulonephritis. Kidney International. Supplement. 2012;**2**:139-274

[23] Johnson JP, Moore J Jr, Austin HA 3rd, et al. Therapy of anti-glomerular basement membrane antibody disease: Analysis of prognostic significance of clinical, pathologic and treatment factors. Medicine (Baltimore). 1985;**64**(4):219

[24] Cui Z, Zhao J, Jia XY, et al. Anti-glomerular basement membrane disease: Outcomes of different therapeutic regimens in a large single-center Chinese cohort study. Medicine (Baltimore). 2011;**90**(5):303-311. DOI: 10.1097/MD.0b013e31822f6f68

[25] Shah Y, Mohiuddin A, Sluman C, et al. Rituximab in anti-glomerular basement membrane disease. QJM. 2012;**105**:195-197. DOI: 10.1016/j.jaut.2015.04.003

[26] Syeda UA, Singer NG, Magrey M. Anti-glomerular basement membrane antibody disease treated with rituximab: A case based review. Seminars in Arthritis and Rheumatism. 2013;**42**:567-572. DOI: 10.1016/j.semarthrit.2012.10.007

[27] Levy JB, Turner AN, Rees AJ, et al. Long-term outcome of anti-glomerular basement membrane antibody disease treated with plasma exchange and immunosuppression. Annals of Internal Medicine. 2001;**134**:1033-1042

[28] Yang R, Hellmark T, Zhao J, et al. Levels of epitope-specific autoantibodies correlate with renal damage in anti-GBM disease. Nephrology, Dialysis, Transplantation. 2009;**24**: 1838-1844. DOI: 10.1093/ndt/gfn761

[29] Jayne DR, Marshall PD, Jones SJ, Lockwood CM. Autoantibodies to GBM and neutrophil cytoplasm in rapidly progressive glomerulonephritis. Kidney International. 1990;**37**(3): 965

[30] McAdoo SP, Pusey CD. Anti-glomerular basement membrane disease. Clinical Journal of the American Society of Nephrology. 2017;**12**(7):1162-1172. DOI: 10.2215/CJN.01380217

[31] Browne G, Brown PA, Tomson CR, et al. Retransplantation in Alport post-transplant anti-GBM disease. Kidney International. 2004;**65**:675-681

[32] Savige J, Gregory M, Gross O, et al. Expert guidelines for the management of Alport syndrome and thin basement membrane nephropathy. Journal of the American Society of Nephrology. 2013;**24**:364-375

[33] Brouet JC, Clauvel JP, Danon F, Kleinc M, Seligmann M. Biologic and clinical significance of cryoglobulins. A report of 86 cases. The American Journal of Medicine. 1974;**57**:775-788

[34] Gorevic PD, Kassab HJ, Levo Y, et al. Mixed cryoglobulinemia: Clinical aspects and long-term follow-up of 40 patients. The American Journal of Medicine. 1980;**69**:287Y308

[35] Morra E. Cryoglobulinemia ASH education book. Hematology. American Society of Hematology. Education Program. 2005;**2005**(1):368Y372

[36] Terrier B, Karras A, Kahn JE, et al. The spectrum of type I cryoglobulinemia vasculitis: New insights based on 64 cases. Medicine (Baltimore). 2013;**92**(2):61-68. DOI: 10.1097/MD.0b013e318288925c

[37] Saadoun D, Sellam J, Ghillani-Dalbin P, Crecel R, Piette JC, Cacoub P. Increased risks of lymphoma and death among patients with non-hepatitis C virus-related mixed cryoglobulinemia. Archives of Internal Medicine. 2006;**166**(19):2101-2108

[38] Couser WG. Basic and translational concepts of immune-mediated glomerular diseases. Journal of the American Society of Nephrology. 2012;**23**:381-399. DOI: 10.1681/ASN.2011030304

[39] Roccatello D, Isidoro C, Mazzucco G, et al. Role of monocytes in cryoglobulinemia-associated nephritis. *Kidney International*. 1993;**43**(5):1150-1155

[40] Puri TS, Quigg RJ. The many effects of complement C3- and C5-binding proteins in renal injury. Seminars in Nephrology. 2007;**27**:321-337

[41] Trendelenburg M, Fossati-Jimack L, Cortes-Hernandez J, et al. The role of complement in cryoglobulin-induced immune complex glomerulonephritis. Journal of Immunology. 2005;**175**(10):6909-6914

[42] Pickering M, Cook HT. Complement and glomerular disease: New insights. Current Opinion in Nephrology and Hypertension. 2011;**20**:271-277. DOI: 10.1097/MNH.0b013e328345848b

[43] Gesualdo L, Grandaliano G, Ranieri E, et al. Monocyte recruitment in cryoglobuline membranoproliferative glomerulonephritis: A pathogenetic role for monocyte chemotactic peptide-1. Kidney International. 1997;**51**:155-163

[44] Reininger L, Berney T, Shibata T, et al. Cryoglobulinemia induced by a murine IgG3 rheumatoid factor: Skin vasculitis and glomerulonephritis arise from distinct pathogenic mechanisms. Proceedings of the National Academy of Sciences of the United States of America. 1990;**87**(24):1038-1042

[45] Cacoub P, Ghillani P, Revelen R, et al. Anti-endothelial cell auto-antibodies in hepatitis C virus mixed cryoglobulinemia. Journal of Hepatology. 1999;**31**:598-603

[46] McMurray RW. Hepatitis C-associated autoimmune disorders. Rheumatic Diseases Clinics of North America. 1998;**24**:353-374

[47] Sansonno D, Lauletta G, Nisi L, et al. Non enveloped HCV core protein as constitutive antigen of cold-precipitable immune complexes in type II mixed cryoglobulinaemia. Clinical and Experimental Immunology. 2003;**133**:275-282

[48] Sansonno D, Tucci FA, Ghebrehiwet B, et al. Role of the receptor for the globular domain of C1q protein in the pathogenesis of hepatitis C virus-related cryoglobulin vascular damage. Journal of Immunology. 2009;**183**:6013-6020. DOI: 10.4049/jimmunol.0902038

[49] Smith KD, Alpers CE. Pathogenic mechanisms in membranoproliferative glomerulonephritis. Current Opinion in Nephrology and Hypertension. 2005;**14**:396-403

[50] Quartuccio L, Fabris M, Salvin S, et al. Bone marrow B-cell clonal expansion in type II mixed cryoglobulinaemia: Association with nephritis. Rheumatology (Oxford, England). 2007;**46**(11):1657-1661

[51] Sansonno D, Lauletta G, Montrone M, et al. Hepatitis C virus RNA and core protein in kidney glomerular and tubular structures isolated with laser capture microdissection. Clinical and Experimental Immunology. 2005;**140**(3):498-506

[52] Landau DA, Saadoun D, Halfon P, et al. Relapse of hepatitis C virus-associated mixed cryoglobulinemia vasculitis in patients with sustained viral response. Arthritis and Rheumatism. 2008;**58**(2):604-611. DOI: 10.1002/art.23305

[53] Kaplanski G, Maisonobe T, Marin V, et al. Vascular cell adhesion molecule-1 (VCAM-1) plays a central role in the pathogenesis of severe forms of vasculitis due to hepatitis C-associated mixed cryoglobulinemia. Journal of Hepatology. 2005;**42**:334-340

[54] Ferri C, Sebastiani M, Giuggioli D, et al. Mixed cryoglobulinemia: Demographic, clinical, and serologic features and survival in 231 patients. Seminars in Arthritis and Rheumatism. 2004;**33**(6):355-374

[55] Terrier B, Krastinova E, Marie I, et al. Management of noninfectious mixed cryoglobulinemia vasculitis: Data from 242 cases included in the CryoVas survey. Blood. 2012;**119**:5996-6004. DOI: 10.1182/blood-2011-12-396028

[56] Terrier B, Carrat F, Krastinova E, et al. Prognostic factors of survival in patients with noninfectious mixed cryoglobulinaemia vasculitis: Data from 242 cases included in the CryoVas survey. Annals of the Rheumatic Diseases. 2013;**72**(3):374-380. DOI: 10.1136/annrheumdis-2012-201405

[57] Ragab G, Hussein MA. Vasculitic syndromes in hepatitis C virus: A review. Journal of Advanced Research. 2017;**8**:99-111. DOI: 10.1016/j.jare.2016.11.002

[58] Terrier B, Semoun O, Saadoun D, et al. Prognostic factors in patients with hepatitis C virus infection and systemic vasculitis. Arthritis and Rheumatism. 2011;**63**:1748-1757. DOI: 10.1002/art.30319

[59] Roccatello D, Fornasieri A, Giachino O, et al. Multicenter study on hepatitis C virus-related cryoglobulinemic glomerulonephritis. American Journal of Kidney Diseases. 2007;**49**(1):69-82

[60] Beddhu S, Bastacky S, Johnson JP. The clinical and morphologic spectrum of renal cryoglobulinemia. Medicine (Baltimore). 2002;**81**(5):398-409

[61] Fischer E, Cerilli LA, Jagger DG. Chapter 5 glomerular diseases-secondary. In: Lager DJ, Abrahams N, editors. Practical Renal Pathology. A Diagnostic Approach. Elsevier Saunders; 2013. eBook ISBN: 9781455737864

[62] De Vita S, Soldano F, Isola M, et al. Preliminary classification criteria for the cryoglobulinemic syndrome. Annals of the Rheumatic Diseases. 2010;**69**(Suppl 3):77

[63] Pietrogrande M, De Vita S, Zignego AL, et al. Recommendations for the management of mixed cryoglobulinemia syndrome in hepatitis C virus-infected patients. Autoimmunity Reviews. 2011;**10**(8):444-454. DOI: 10.1016/j.autrev.2011.01.008

[64] Sneller MC, Hu Z, Langford CA. A randomized controlled trial of rituximab following failure of antiviral therapy for hepatitis C virus-associated cryoglobulinemic vasculitis. Arthritis and Rheumatism. 2012;**64**:835-842. DOI: 10.1002/art.34322

[65] Lake-Bakaar G, Dustin L, McKeating J, et al. Hepatitis C virus and alanine aminotransferase kinetics following B-lymphocyte depletion with rituximab: Evidence for a significant role of humoral immunity in the control of viremia in chronic HCV liver disease. Blood. 2007;**109**(2):845-846

[66] De Vita S, Quartuccio L, Isola M, et al. A randomized controlled trial of rituximab for the treatment of severe cryoglobulinemic vasculitis. Arthritis and Rheumatism. 2012;**64**:843-853. DOI: 10.1002/art.34331

[67] Yeo W, Chan TC, Leung NW, et al. Hepatitis B virus reactivation in lymphoma patients with prior resolved hepatitis B undergoing anticancer therapy with or without rituximab. Journal of Clinical Oncology. 2009;**27**(4):605-611. DOI: 10.1200/JCO.2008.18.0182

[68] Klepfish A, Schattner A, Shvidel L, et al. Successful treatment of aggressive HIVassociated non-Hodgkin's lymphoma with combination chemotherapy, biotherapy with rituximab and HAART: Presentation of a therapeutic option. Leukemia & Lymphoma. 2003;**44**(2):349-351

[69] Terrier B, Marie I, Lacraz A, et al. Non HCV related infectious cryoglobulinemia vasculitis: Results from the French nationwide CryoVas survey and systematic review of the literature. Journal of Autoimmunity. 2015;**65**:74-81. DOI: 10.1016/j.jaut.2015.08.008

[70] Quartuccio L, Soardo G, Romano G, et al. Rituximab treatment for glomerulonephritis in HCV-associated mixed cryoglobulinaemia: Efficacy and safety in the absence of steroids. Rheumatology. 2006;**45**:842-846

[71] Mukhtyar C, Guillevin L, Cid MC, et al. EULAR recommendations for the management of primary small and medium vessel vasculitis. Annals of the Rheumatic Diseases. 2009;**68**:310-317. DOI: 10.1136/ard.2008.088096

[72] Schwartz J, Padmanabhan A, Aqui N, et al. Guidelines on the use of therapeutic apheresis in clinical practice-evidence-based approach from the writing committee of the American Society for Apheresis: The seventh special issue. Journal of Clinical Apheresis. 2016;**31**(3):149-162. DOI: 10.1002/jca.21470

[73] Marinaki S, Drouzas K, Skalioti C, Boletis JN. Chapter 12. Hepatitis B and C in kidney transplantation. In: Allam N, editor. Advances in Treatment of Hepatitis C and B. Croatia: In Tech. DOI: 10.5772/65381

[74] European Association for the Study of the Liver. EASL recommendation on treatment of hepatitis C 2015. Journal of Hepatology. 2015;**63**:199-236. DOI: 10.1016/j.jhep.2015.03.025

[75] Gragnani L, Visentini M, Fognani E, et al. Prospective study of guideline-tailored therapy with direct-acting antivirals for hepatitis C virusassociated mixed cryoglobulinemia. Hepatology. 2016;**64**(5):1473-1482. DOI: 10.1002/hep.28753

[76] Viganò M, Martin P, Cappelletti M, Fabrizi F. HBV associated cryoglobulinemic vasculitis: Remission after antiviral therapy with entecavir. Kidney & Blood Pressure Research. 2014;**39**:65-73. DOI: 10.1159/000355778

[77] Muchtar E, Magen H, Gertz MA. How I treat cryoglobulinemia. Blood. 2017;**129**(3):289-298. DOI: 10.1182/blood-2016-09-719773

[78] Dimopoulos MA, Zervas C, Zomas A, Kiamouris C, Viniou NA, Grigoraki V, Karkantaris C, Mitsouli C, Gika D, Christakis J, Anagnostopoulos N. Treatment of Waldenstrom's macroglobulinemia with rituximab. Journal of Clinical Oncology. 2002;**20**(9):2327-2333. DOI: 10.1200/JCO.2002.09.039

[79] Heberden W. Commentari di Morborium-Historia e Cutatione. London: Payne; 1802

[80] Schoenlein JL. Allgemeine Und Spezielle Pathologie Und Therapie. Etlinger: Wuerzburg. p. 1832

[81] Henoch E. Neunter Abschnitt. Die haemorragische Purpura. Hirschwald; 1874

[82] Pillebout E. Adult Henoch-Schönlein purpura. Presse Médicale. 2008;**37**(12):1773-1778. DOI: 10.1016/j.lpm.2008.05.002. [Article in French]

[83] Gardner-Medwin JM, Dolezalova P, Cummins C, et al. Incidence of Henoch-Schönlein purpura, Kawasaki disease, and rare vasculitides in children of different ethnic origins. Lancet. 2002;**360**(9341):1197-1202

[84] Trapani S, Micheli A, Grisolia F, et al. Henoch-Schonlein purpura in childhood: Epidemiological and clinical analysis of 150 cases over a 5-year period and review of literature. Seminars in Arthritis and Rheumatism. 2005;**35**:143-153

[85] Julian BA, Wyatt RJ, Waldo FB, et al. Immunological studies of IgA nephropathy: Familial and racial aspects. Advances in Experimental Medicine and Biology. 1987;**216B**:1489-1498

[86] Kiryluk K, Novak J. The genetics and immunobiology of IgA nephropathy. The Journal of Clinical Investigation. 2014;**124**:2325-2332. DOI: 10.1172/JCI74475

[87] Pankhurst T, Savage CO, Gordon C, et al. Malignancy is increased in ANCA-associated vasculitis. Rheumatology (Oxford, England). 2004;**43**(12):1532-1535

[88] Pillebout E, Thervet E, Hill G, et al. Henoch-Schönlein Purpura in adults: Outcome and prognostic factors. Journal of the American Society of Nephrology. 2002;**13**(5):1271-1278

[89] Zickerman AM, Allen AC, Talwar V, et al. IgA myeloma presenting as Henoch-Schönlein purpura with nephritis. American Journal of Kidney Diseases. 2000;**36**(3):E19

[90] Ergin S, Sanli Erdoğan B, Turgut H, et al. Relapsing Henoch-Schönlein purpura in an adult patient associated with hepatitis B virus infection. The Journal of Dermatology. 2005;**32**(10):839-834

[91] Chave T, Neal C, Camp R. Henoch-Schönlein purpura following hepatitis B vaccination. The Journal of Dermatological Treatment. 2003;**14**(3):179-181

[92] Borrás-Blasco J, Enriquez R, Amoros F, et al. Henoch-Schönlein purpura associated with clarithromycin. Case report and review of literature. International Journal of Clinical Pharmacology and Therapeutics. 2003;**41**(5):213-216. Erratum in: Int J Clin Pharmacol Ther. 2003;41(9):420

[93] Rigante D, Castellazzi L, Bosco A, et al. Is there a crossroad between infections, genetics, and Henoch-Schönlein purpura? Autoimmunity Reviews. 2013;**12**(10):1016-1021. DOI: 10.1016/j.autrev.2013.04.003

[94] Wyatt RJ, Julian BA. IgA nephropathy. The New England Journal of Medicine. 2013;**368**(25):2402-2414. DOI: 10.1056/nejmra1206793

[95] Saulsbury FT. Henoch-Schönlein purpura in children: Report of 100 patients and review of the literature. Medicine. 1999;**78**:395-409

[96] Magro CM, Crowson AN. A clinical and histologic study of 37 cases of immunoglobulin associated vasculitis. The American Journal of Dermatopathology. 1999;**21**(3):234-240

[97] Calvino MC, Llorca J, Garcia-Porrua C, et al. Henoch-Schönlein purpura in children from northwestern Spain: A 20-year epidemiologic and clinical study. Medicine. 2001;**80**: 279-290

[98] Yang YH, Yu HH, Chiang BL. The diagnosis and classification of Henoch-Schönlein purpura: An updated review. Autoimmunity Reviews. 2014;**13**(4-5):355-358. DOI: 10.1016/j.autrev.2014.01.031

[99] Audemard-Verger A, Pillebout E, Guillevin L, et al. IgA vasculitis (Henoch-Shönlein purpura) in adults: Diagnostic and therapeutic aspects. Autoimmunity Reviews. 2015;**14**(7): 579-585. DOI: 10.1016/j.autrev.2015.02.003

[100] Esaki M, Matsumoto T, Nakamura S, et al. GI involvement in Henoch-Schönlein purpura. Gastrointestinal Endoscopy. 2002;**56**(6):920-923

[101] Kellerman PS. Henoch-Schönlein purpura in adults. American Journal of Kidney Diseases. 2006;**48**(6):1009-1016

[102] Haas M. IgA nephropathy and Henoch-Schoenlein purpura nephritis. In: Jennette JC, Olsen JL, Schwartz MM, Silva FG, editors. Heptinstall's Pathology of the Kidney. 6th ed. Philadelphia: Lippincott Williams & Wilkins; 2007. pp. 423-486

[103] Working Group of the International IgA Nephropathy Network and the Renal Pathology Society, Cattran DC, Coppo R, Cook HT, et al. The Oxford classification of IgA nephropathy: Rationale, clinicopathological correlations, and classification. Kidney International. 2009;**76**(5):534-545

[104] Coppo R, Mazzucco G, Cagnoli L, et al. Long-term prognosis of Henoch-Schönlein nephritis in adults and children. Italian Group of Renal Immunopathology Collaborative Study on Henoch-Schönlein purpura. Nephrology, Dialysis, Transplantation. 1997;**12**(11):2277-2283

[105] Blanco R, Martínez-Taboada VM, Rodríguez-Valverde V, et al. Henoch-Schönlein purpura in adulthood and childhood: Two different expressions of the same syndrome. Arthritis and Rheumatism. 1997;**40**(5):859-864

[106] Rauta V, Törnroth T, Grönhagen-Riska C. Henoch-Schoenlein nephritis in adults-clinical features and outcomes in finnish patients. Clinical Nephrology. 2002;**58**(1):1-8

[107] Pillebout E, Alberti C, Guillevin L, et al. Addition of cyclophosphamide to steroids provides no benefit compared with steroids alone in treating adult patients with severe Henoch Schönlein Purpura. Kidney International. 2010;**78**(5):495-502. DOI: 10.1038/ki.2010.150

[108] Floege J, Eitner F. Current therapy for IgA nephropathy. Journal of the American Society of Nephrology. 2011;**22**(10):1785-1794. DOI: 10.1681/ASN.2011030221

[109] Rauen T, Eitner F, Fitzner C, et al. Intensive supportive care plus immunosuppression in IgA nephropathy. The New England Journal of Medicine. 2015;**373**(23):2225-2236. DOI: 10.1056/nejmoa1415463

[110] Gutierrez E, Gonzalez E, Hernandez E, et al. Factors that determine an incomplete recovery of renal function in macrohematuria-induced acute renal failure of IgA nephropathy. Clinical Journal of the American Society of Nephrology. 2007;**2**:51-57

[111] Harper L, Ferreira MA, Howie AJ, et al. Treatment of vasculitic IgA nephropathy. Journal of Nephrology. 2000;**13**:360-366

[112] Pankhurst T, Lepenies J, Nightingale P, et al. Vasculitic IgA nephropathy: Prognosis and outcome. Nephron. Clinical Practice. 2009;**112**:c16-c24. DOI: 10.1159/000210570

[113] Lai KN, Lai FM, Ho CP, et al. Corticosteroid therapy in IgA nephropathy with nephrotic syndrome: A long-term controlled trial. Clinical Nephrology. 1986;**26**:174-180

[114] Padeh S, Passwell JH. Successful treatment of chronic Henoch–Schonlein purpura with colchicine and aspirin. The Israel Medical Association Journal. 2000;**2**(6):482-483

[115] Papandreou T, Dürken M, Goebeler M, et al. Chronic recalcitrant Henoch–Schönlein purpura: Successful treatment with dapsone. European Journal of Dermatology. 2010;**20**:639-640. DOI: 10.1684/ejd.2010.1009

[116] Wu SH, Liao PY, Chen XQ, et al. Add-on therapy with montelukast in the treatment of Henoch–Schönlein purpura. Pediatrics International. 2014;**56**(3):315-322. DOI: 10.1111/ped.12271

[117] Ronkainen J, Koskimies O, Ala-Houhala M, et al. Early prednisone therapy in Henoch-Schönlein purpura: A randomized, double–blind, placebo-controlled trial. The Journal of Pediatrics. 2006;**149**:241-247

Section 3

Relevant Pathogenic and Clinical Updates

Chapter 4

p53 and Vascular Dysfunction: MicroRNA in Endothelial Cells

Munekazu Yamakuchi, Sushil Panta and
Teruto Hashiguchi

Additional information is available at the end of the chapter

http://dx.doi.org/10.5772/intechopen.75461

Abstract

In many cancer cells, p53 gene is mutated and accumulated, which is considered as a mechanistical target of tumorigenesis. The role of p53 in non-cancerous cells has been focused on, since p53 activation diversely affects as human diseases, including vascular dysfunctions. p53 regulates vascular events, including vascular inflammation and senescence as well as cardiac dysfunction. Many researchers also have paid attention to the role of noncoding RNAs (ncRNAs), especially small-sized microRNAs (miRNAs) for the last decade and their noble biological cellular functions have been discovered. miRNAs expressed in endothelial cells (endothelial miRNAs) have been shown to control vascular events. Firstly, the importance of p53 in a variety of vascular events, such as vascular inflammation and senescence, are summarized. Secondly, the way to regulate miRNAs by p53 and the involvement of miRNAs on p53 function are demonstrated. Finally, several endothelial miRNAs that have important roles are focused on. The aim of this chapter is to understand the role of p53 in vascular diseases in the view of endothelial cell biology and the contribution of miRNAs related to p53.

Keywords: endothelial cells, miRNAs, p53, Dicer, Drosha

1. Introduction

1.1. p53 overview

p53 is one of well-known tumor suppressor protein and plays crucial roles in inhibiting tumor progression [1]. Tumor suppression by p53 might be carried out mostly through genotoxic stress, however, recent studies revealed that p53 is activated by oncogene activation, oxidized lipoproteins, and hypoxic condition [2]. In general, p53 is rapidly degraded by the interaction with MDM2 and these stimuli increase p53 levels and activate antiproliferative or proapoptotic responses via downstream signaling molecules [3]. The structure of p53 consists of amino terminal transactivation domain linked to the DNA-binding domain by proline-rich region (**Figure 1**) [4]. The DNA-binding domain on the other end is bound to the tetramerization domain by another proline-rich residue and this tetramerization domain is linked to carboxyl terminus [5]. The core domain (residue 94–312) is naturally unstable and is prone to have mutation [6, 7]. Once bound to the DNA, the whole structure closes around the DNA double helix. The whole process is facilitated by flexible proline-rich region between the core and the tetramerization domain [5]. Although the expression of p53 is in lower level during normal condition, upon activation, p53 increases its level along with the increase of its half-life [8] and gets translocated to the nucleus [9]. p53 is activated mainly by any signals that could damage the DNA [10]. Further p53 undergoes phosphorylation, acetylation, methylation, ubiquitination or SUMOylation to exert its respective activity [11]. p53 interacts with p300/CBP to get acetylated which stimulates the binding of p53 to the DNA, however, p53 requires only p300 but not CBP for the well-known G1 arrest [12]. Two members of p53 family, p73 and p63, are also involved in this p53 world [13], which are not mentioned in this chapter. Regulation and function of p53 in cancer really become complex.

1.2. p53 and endothelial cells

In the complex network of cellular signaling, p53 is a transcription factor that plays an important role in controlling angiogenesis and it is a hub for cellular signaling [14]. p53 itself controls angiogenesis by taking cells under apoptosis or by downregulating mediators of angiogenesis [15]. The role of p53 in vasculature is the same as the other tissues, including cell cycle, apoptosis, senescence, and angiogenesis.

Mice genetically deleted p53 can develop normally, however, these p53 knockout mice had spontaneous tumors [16]. Conditional knockout of p53 in endothelial cells improves angiogenesis of hindlimb ischemia mice model [17]. When mice were fed diet with high calorie, p53 expression increased in endothelial cells [18]. High calorie diet impaired the activation of endothelial nitric oxide synthase (eNOS), which was restored in endothelial p53 disruption. Knockdown of p53 in endothelial cells increased the expression of eNOS and thrombomodulin in vitro [19]. Therefore, accumulating evidence suggested that p53 is one of the key transcriptional factors to regulate endothelial cell function.

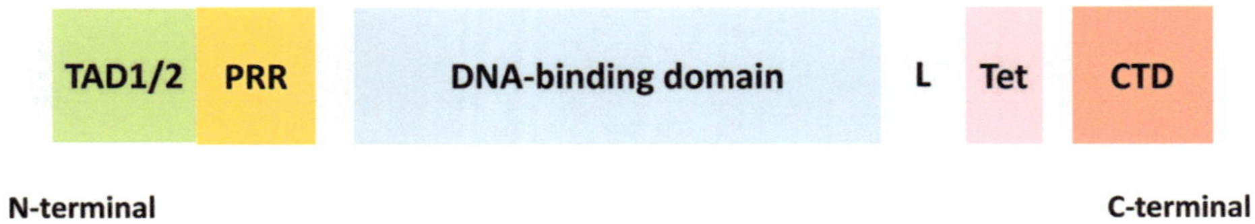

Figure 1. Linear structure of p53. p53 consists of 393 amino acid sequence. The protein is divided into the following domains. The transcriptional activation domain 1/2 (TAD1/2), DNA-binding domain, and the tetramerization domains (Tet) are lysine-rich basic C-terminal domain (CTD). PRR, proline-rich region; L, the linker region; Tet, tetramerization domains.

2. p53 and vascular function

Normal cells including endothelial cells keep p53 levels quite low. Low grade upregulation of p53 is not apoptotic but it is engaged in other functions like inhibition of endothelial cell migration through downregulation of beta-3 integrin [20] and inhibition of cell survival by causing reversible cell cycle arrest [21]. The modulation of p53 varies vascular function, such as vascular inflammation, senescence, and remodeling.

2.1. Vascular inflammation

Vascular inflammation leads to form atherosclerotic lesions, in which many cells are orchestrating [22]. Role of p53 in atherosclerosis has been investigated by many researchers. Guevara et al. performed the experiments using double knockout mice with apolipoprotein E (apoE) and p53. This $apoE^{-/-}$, $p53^{-/-}$ double knockout mice fed with high fat diet showed significant increase of bulky, hypercellular lesion in aorta, suggesting that p53 is involved in atherosclerotic change [23]. van Vlijmen et al. demonstrated that the role of p53 in subendothelial macrophages is one of the major components of atherosclerosis [24]. This study indicated that deficiency of p53 in macrophage increased atherosclerotic lesions. Oxidative stress induces p53 accumulation in human macrophage, which is prevented by nitric oxide (NO) [25]. NO blocked the secretion of von Willebrand factor in endothelial cells and inhibited vascular inflammation [26]. The molecular mechanism by which p53 regulates atherosclerosis has been aggressively investigated.

2.2. Senescence

Aging is an independent risk factor for atherosclerosis-related diseases and impairment of vascular function is involved in systematic senescence. The molecular difference between senescence and cell death is not an easy question. Disturbed blood flow (d-flow) causes atherosclerosis. Heo KS et al. identified protein kinase zeta (PKC zeta) as a d-flow-activated protein in endothelial cells [27]. d-Flow promotes endothelial cells apoptosis through p53 SUMOylation. Apoptosis in aortic endothelial cells by d-flow decreased in $p53^{-/-}$ mice compared to wild type mice. Endothelial cells constitutively express Nox2 and Nox4, two important isoforms of catalytic subunit of NADPH, which are a major source of reactive oxygen species. Nox2 especially affects endothelial cell cycle arrest and cell death by modulating p53 and p21cip1 [28]. In turn, cellular senescence is a stress-induced phenomenon as well. Senescent cells delay or lose the ability to proliferate. In endothelial cells, hydrogen peroxide or frequent passage induces cellular senescence via p53 and NAD-dependent deacetylase sirtuin-1 (SIRT1) [29]. The expression of endothelial SIRT-1 is reduced during aging process [30, 31]. Reduced SIRT-1 in endothelial cells accumulates genomic instability, resulting in p53 activation and promoting more senescence [32, 33]. AMPK and mTOR signaling is thought to be important for endothelial aging [34, 35]. These molecules are also connected to p53 signals, suggesting p53 as a key regulator of senescence of endothelial cells.

2.3. Vascular and heart remodeling

Vascular remodeling is a process of structural change of vascular walls, involving changes of cellular function, including growth and death. In this process, p53 is an important player.

Chronic hypoxia promotes pulmonary vascular remodeling, causing pulmonary hypertension. Mizuno S et al. demonstrated that p53 suppress hypoxia-induced pulmonary arterial remodeling and pulmonary arterial smooth muscle cell proliferation [36]. Kruppel-like factor 4 (KLF4) controls vascular smooth muscle cell proliferation through p53 induction [37]. Cardiac remodeling and development occur during embryogenesis but stop in postnatal life due to the reduction of the genes responsible for cell cycle progression and growth factors [38, 39]. For remodeling, new cardiomyocytes are derived for pre-existing cardiomyocytes. The rate of the pre-existing cells differentiation is very low (less than 1% per year) and it decreases with age [40] and lesser then 50% of the cells are replaced during a lifespan [41]. One important molecule for cardiomyocyte division is survivin [42]. Downregulation of survivin contributes to cardiac development in spinal muscular atrophy mice model [43]. Survivin is negatively regulated by p53. Survivin expression was downregulated at mRNA and protein level by p53 through histone acetylation. While overexpression of survivin inhibited p53-induced apoptosis [44]. One of MAPK, p38, has been shown to be an important molecule that negatively regulates cell cycle in cardiomyocyte cell [45]. Treatment with FGF1 and p38 inhibitor enhanced heart regeneration by increasing cardiomyocyte proliferation and angiogenesis [46]. Repression of cyclin D1 result into downregulation of cardiac cell proliferation [47] and C reactive protein, besides downregulating cyclin D1 has been shown to accumulate and phosphorylate p53 which leads to cell cycle arrest [48]. Since p53 controls actin cytoskeleton through mechanoresponsive molecules, remodeling may be processing via p53 in mechanical environment-dependent manner.

3. p53 and miRNA in endothelial cells

3.1. miRNA overview: general information

MicroRNAs (miRNAs) are small noncoding RNAs (about 20–24 nucleotides in length) that controls gene expressions mainly by binding to 3′ untranslated region (3′ UTR) of their messenger RNAs (mRNAs). The biogenesis of miRNAs in animals is very unique (**Figure 2**). Primary miRNAs (pri-miRNAs) are transcribed from miRNA-encoding genes. miRNAs are encoded in any place; some are located on protein-coding region, and some are in noncoding region or intron [49]. The pri-miRNAs are cleaved into hairpin-structured small size RNAs (precursor miRNAs; pre-miRNAs) by microprocessor complex containing RNase III, Drosha and DiGeorge critical region 8 (DGCR8) [50]. Exportin 5 (XPO5) and Ran-GTP transported pre-miRNAs into the cytoplasm from the nucleus, then pre-miRNAs are cleaved in double-stranded smaller RNAs (miRNA duplexes) by another RNase III, Dicer [51]. One of the strand (mature miRNAs) are incorporated into miRNA-induced silencing complex containing Argonaute 2 (Ago2) and transactivation response RNA-binding protein (TRBP) in human and these miRNAs are ready to bind to target mRNAs [52] (**Figure 2**).

How do miRNAs inhibit the expression of target protein? In general, miRNAs use two ways of silencing: repression of translation and mRNA decay [53]. The seed sequence of miRNA (2–7 position from 5′ end) can bind to 3′UTR of target mRNA with incomplete match in animals. This miRNA-mRNA binding leads to repress the translation or destroy miRNA [54]. More than 60% of protein is regulated by miRNAs in human [55, 56]. Therefore, miRNAs are involved in modifying ubiquitous cellular functions.

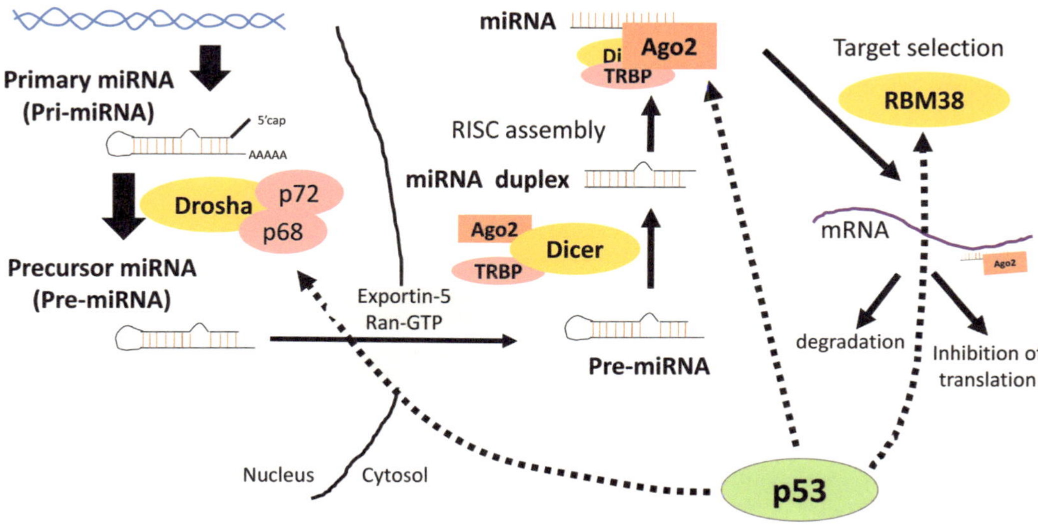

Figure 2. p53 regulation of miRNA biogenesis.

3.2. miRNAs and p53

The relationship between miRNA and cancer was first described by Calin GA et al. in 2002. They described downregulation of miR-15a and miR-16-1 in B cell chronic lymphocytic leukemia patients [57]. miRNAs associated with cancer are called 'oncomiR', which have been identified in many types of cancer [58]. Some oncomiRs decrease in cancerous tissue. In contrast, increased oncomiRs are also found in cancer, which in case inhibit tumor suppressor genes, following the proliferation of cancer cells. The proto-oncogene c-Myc is a transcriptional factor and dysregulation of c-Myc was found in many cancers. The studies for regulation of transcriptional factors by miRNAs have been started since O'Donnell et al. identified mir-17-92, a polycistronic miRNA transcript that yields six individual miRNA components, as c-Myc-regulated miRNAs in human B cell line [59]. It was not hard to assume that the next target of 'transcription factors' regulating miRNAs in cancer was p53.

3.3. Direct regulation of miRNAs by p53

In 2007, several articles about p53 regulation of miRNAs have been published independently from different research groups. All these studies revealed that p53 upregulated the expression of miR-34 family in different cells [60–64]. The miR-34 family comprises three members (**Figure 4C**). miR-34a is generated from the large transcript on chromosome 1p36 and miR-34b and miR-34c are generated from bicistronic transcript on chromosome 11q23 [65]. Though the expression levels of miR-34a, -34b, and -34c were not consistent in non-small cell lung cancers (NSCLCs) compared to the adjacent normal tissue, lower expressions of three miR-34 family members are lower in many cancer cell lines; H1299 (lung cancer), MCF-7 (breast cancer), U-2OS (osteosarcoma), HCT116 (colon cancer), and many pancreatic cancer cell lines such as PANC1 [60, 64]. In addition to cancer, p53 regulates miR-34 family in non-cancerous cells, such as mouse embryonic fibroblasts (MEFs) and human fetal lung fibroblasts (IMR-90 cells) [63].

Forced expression of miR-34 family induce growth arrest and apoptosis in a variety of cell lines, whatever cancers or non-cancerous cells [62]. A lot of target genes of miR-34 family have been identified, including cyclin E2 (CCNE2), cyclin-dependent kinase 4 (CDK4) and the hepatocyte growth factor receptor (MET), B cell CLL/lymphoma 2 (BCL2), baculoviral IAP repeat-containing 3 (BIRC3), and decoy receptor 3 (DcR3 also known as TNFRSF6B). Many miRNAs directly induced by p53 have been identified in cancer cell lines. As described above, miR-34a might be the most fascinating one. Among these p53-induced miRNAs, several miRNAs that affect endothelial function are demonstrated in **Figure 5A**.

3.3.1. miR-34 family

The expression of miR-34 family, which consists of miR-34a, -34b, and -34c are induced by p53 activation [60, 64]. In many cancers, miR-34a-promoted apoptosis as described in the previous section. In primary normal human cells, miR-34 family can change cellular senescence. A series of miRNAs, including miR-34a, were upregulated in hydrogen peroxide-induced premature senescence in human fibroblasts [66]. There are two human p53 isoforms, p53 beta which lacks C-terminal oligomerization domain and delta133 p53 which lacks N-terminal transactivation and proline-rich domains. Human fibroblasts (MBC-5 and WI-38) at early passage had many delta133 p53 but not p53 beta. In contrast, p53 beta expressed well in fibroblasts at late passage. In fibroblasts, miR-34a control replicative cellular senescence and delta133 p53 repressed miR-34a expression, extending cellular replicative lifespan [67].

Aging of endothelial cells is one of the factors for cardiovascular diseases. miR-34a, expressed relatively higher in late-passage endothelial cells, modulated endothelial cell survival and senescence [30]. Overexpression of miR-34a triggers endothelial senescence mainly by blocking SIRT1. In mice, miR-34a expression also increases in heart and spleen from older ones. Endothelial progenitor cells (EPCs) are essential for many physiological processes such as wound healing. miR-34a impairs EPC-mediated angiogenesis by increasing the number of senescent EPC probably through SIRT1 inhibition [68]. SIRT1, the major target of miR-34a, was known to deacetylate p53. Activation of p53 increased miR-34a expression, which inhibit SIRT1 expression, causing accumulation of acetylated p53. Acetylated p53 induces cell cycle arrest and apoptosis, and this increase of p53 activity induced more miR-34a expression. This suggests that p53 – miR-34a – SIRT1 works as a positive feedback loop (**Figure 3B**) [69].

Notch signaling has crucial role in artery-vein differentiation, blood vessel sprouting, and branching. Dysregulation of Notch signaling causes cardiovascular diseases [70]. miR-34a could regulate Notch signaling pathway in vascular inflammation. In the case of placental dysfunction, miR-34a exacerbated vascular endothelial inflammation via suppression of regulator of calcineurin 1 (RCAN1) [71]. Shear stress is one of the central regulators of endothelial inflammatory responses. The expression of miR-34a decreased by anti-inflammatory physiological high shear stress, in turn, inflammatory oscillatory shear stress-induced miR-34a expression in endothelial cells [72]. Increased miR-34a promoted acetylation of NF-kB p65 subunit (Lys310) by downregulating SIRT1, which lead to upregulate vascular cell adhesion molecule-1 (VCAM-1) and intercellular adhesion molecule-1 (ICAM-1) protein expression. miR-34a also contributed to shear stress-induced EPC differentiation through a novel target Forkhead box j2 (Foxj2) [73]. The important molecules targeting by endothelial miR-34a are listed in **Figure 3A**.

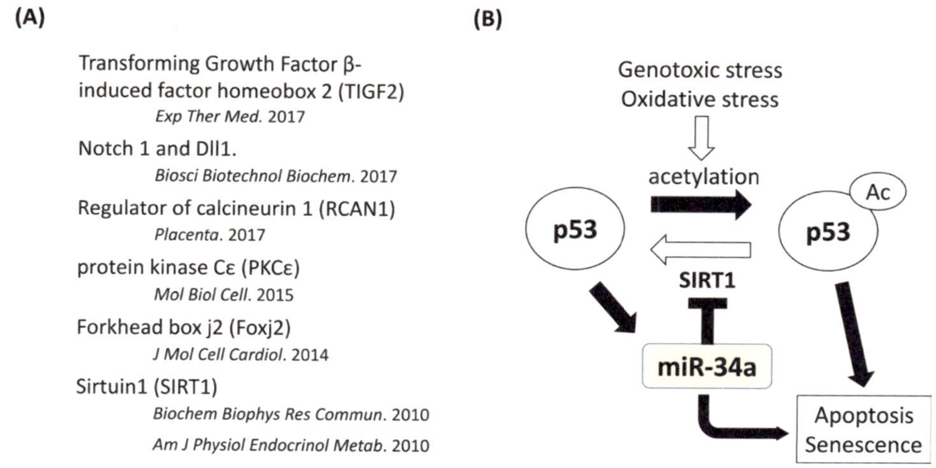

Figure 3. The role of miR-34a in regulating endothelial functions. (A) miR-34a target in endothelial cells. (B) miR-34a – p53 feedback loop.

3.3.2. miR-103 and miR-107

P53 positively regulates expressions of miR-103 and miR-107 in colorectal cancer cell lines [74]. miR-107 is encoded within an intron of the gene for pantothenate kinase enzyme 1, PANK1, while miR-103 is produced from primary miRNAs which are on miR-103-1 and miR-103-2 locus (within introns of PANK2 and PANK3, respectively) (**Figure 4A**). The seed sequences of miR-103 and miR-107 are the same, therefore, these miRNAs should have similar function [75]. miR-103 and miR-107 (miR-103/107) were originally recognized as a key regulator of metabolism and a hypoxia responsible miRNA [76]. The levels of miR-103/107 increased in liver of obese mice, ob/ob mice and diet-induced obese (DIO) mice, and knockdown of miR-103/107 improved insulin sensitivity [77]. Caveolin-1 was one of miR-103/107 targets that altered the level of insulin receptor on lipid rafts.

miR-103/107 also affected angiogenesis as members of hypoxia-responsive microRNAs (HRMs) induced by HIF1α under hypoxia in endothelial cells [78, 79]. The crucial proteins for miRNA biogenesis, Dicer-1 and Ago-1, were identified as miR-107 and miR-103/107 targets, respectively. In both cases, miR-107 provided translational de-suppression of vascular endothelial growth factor (VEGF) mRNA and increased VEGF expression. AGO1 levels regulated by miR-103/107 were associated with higher survival rate in human hepatocellular carcinoma [78]. Antagomir-107 decreased the number of capillaries in ischemic boundary zone after permanent middle cerebral artery occlusion (pMCAO) in rats, which was caused by miR-107 – Dicer-1 – VEGF axis [79].

In sepsis, miR-107 plays an important role in endothelial cells. One of the major complications of sepsis is the development of acute kidney injury (AKI) [80]. Septic AKI activates renal endothelial cells and leads to inflammation and breakdown of endothelial barrier in kidney [81]. Wang et al. isolated circulating endothelial cells (CECs) from septic AKI patients and prepared CEC-conditioned media. Human tubule epithelial cells (HK2 cells) treated with this CEC-conditioned media became more apoptotic, which was regulated by miR-107 [82].

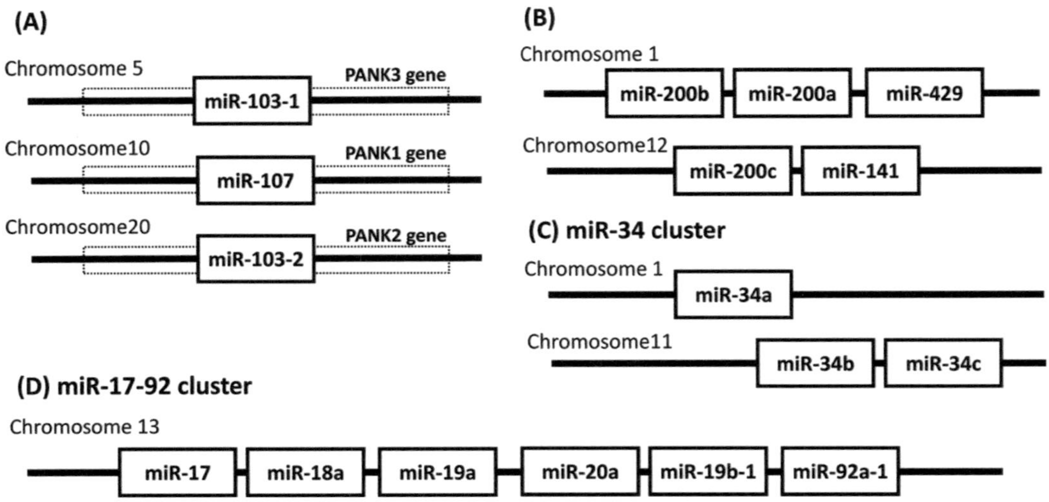

Figure 4. Scheme of miRNA cluster (miR-103/107, miR-200/141, miR-34, and miR-17-92). (A) miR-103/107 cluster. (B) miR-200/141 cluster. (C) miR-34 cluster. (D) miR-17-92 cluster.

In brain, miR-107 is enriched in neuron and the expression of miR-107 decreased in cerebral cortical gray matter of patients with Alzheimer's disease (AD) [83]. The authors demonstrated that beta-site amyloid precursor protein-cleaving enzyme 1 (BACE1) was identified as a miR-107 target. The cerebrovascular deposition of the amyloid beta protein, the key molecule in Alzheimer's disease, causes the disruption of blood-brain barrier (BBB) and brain microvascular endothelial cell dysfunction [84]. Another studies showed that miR-107 prevented amyloid beta-induced endothelial cells dysfunction by targeting endophilin-1 [85]. In a transgenic mouse model of AD, miR-107 expression in brain was lower compared to that in wild type mice [86]. Cofilin, which maintains the structure and function of cytoskeleton, was proved to be regulated by miR-107 in this mouse model. These data from AD patients and mice model suggest that relative high level of miR-107 in neurons and endothelial cells might negatively control the onset and progression of AD.

3.3.3. miR-143/145

miR-143 and miR-145 forms a bicistronic cluster (miR-143/145 cluster) in 5q33.1. The miR-143/145 cluster has been recognized as a tumor suppressor [87]. In cervical cancer, overexpression of Musashi RNA-binding protein 2 (MSI-2) correlated with poor survival. MSI-2 was repressed by p53 regulated miRNAs, miR-143 and miR-107, resulting in the prevention from proliferation and invasion of cervical cancer cells [88]. miR-143 and miR-145 have also potential roles in differentiation of vascular smooth muscle cells [89, 90]. The expression of miR-143/145 cluster decreased in aortic aneurysms and coronary artery diseases [91, 92]. miR-145-5p controls vascular neointimal lesion formation in balloon-injured rat carotid arteries [93]. The expression of miR-145 was upregulated in the lung of bone morphogenetic protein receptor type 2 (BMPR2)-deficient mice and puomonary arterial hypertension (PAH) patients [94]. Deng L. et al. identified transcriptional factors that regulate miR-143 and miR-145 expression in the promoter of miR-143/145 cluster [95]. Each miRNA in this cluster has each function; however, how this cluster or miR-143 and miR145 independently regulated has not been fully understood yet.

Shear stress suppressed angiotensin-converting enzyme (ACE) expression and increased miR-143/145 levels in HUVEC [96]. The authors have shown that shear stress elicited the AMP-activated protein kinase alpha2 (AMPKα2)-dependent phosphorylation of p53 (Serine 15), and that p53 downregulation prevented the shear stress induced decrease in ACE expression. Since overexpression of miR-143/145 decreased ACE expression, AMPKα2 suppresses ACE expression through p53 activation and upregulation of miR-143/145 in EC. AMPKα2 knockout mice showed higher ACE levels and impaired bradykinin-induced vasodilation compared to wild type mice. In streptozotocin-induced diabetes mellitus (DM) mice model, phosphorylation of p53 and miR-143/145 expression increased, leading to the decrease of ACE expression. Therefore, miR-143 and miR-145 may contribute to the vascular events in atherosclerosis and DM.

miR-143 itself has been studied for the role of VSMCs as well as miR-145. The expression of miR-143 decreased in proliferating hemangiomas and miR-143 overexpression suppressed cell viability and proliferation of hemangioma-derived endothelial cells [97]. Bai Y et al. showed that miR-143 is upregulated in the brain microvessels of methamphetamine-treated mice [98]. Knockdown of miR-143 protected brain-blood barrier (BBB) damage-related vascular dysfunction by methamphetamine exposure. They identified an apoptosis inducing molecule, p53 upregulated modulator of apoptosis (PUMA), as a target of miR-143. Since the expression of miR-143 was regulated by p53 and miR-143 decreased PUMA, miR-143 might act for negative feedback of p53 signaling.

3.3.4. *Others: miR-192, miR-200 family, and miR-194*

Dysregulation of redox balance affects vascular homeostasis. Hydrogen peroxide treatment significantly increased miR-192 levels, which were prevented by p53 knockdown in endothelial cells [99]. Overexpression of miR-192 inhibited endothelial cell growth. Another study has shown that miR-200 family and miR-141 were upregulated in HUVEC exposed to hydrogen peroxide and in skeletal muscle in acute hindlimb ischemia mice model [100]. miRNA-200 family consists of two clusters, one encodes miR-200b, miR-200a, and miR-429 from chromosome 1 (1p33.36) and the other has miR-200c and miR-141 from chromosome 2 (12p13.31) (**Figure 4B**). These miRNAs share the similar seed sequence and mostly target the same genes. miR-200 family targets ZEB1 and ZEB2, affecting endothelial cell proliferation and senescence as well as epithelial-mesenchymal transition (EMT). Astrocytes are involved in controlling central nerve system (CNS) damage. During repair process of CNS, astrocytes undergo phenotypic changes into endothelial cells. This astrocyte-endothelial cell transition was modulated by a p53 inducible miRNA, miR-194. Therefore, miR-194 could promote angiogenesis in CNS.

3.4. Regulation of miRNA biogenesis by p53

There are two mechanisms by which p53 regulates miRNA production - control of miRNA transcription and modulation of miRNA maturation. These representative miRNAs regu-

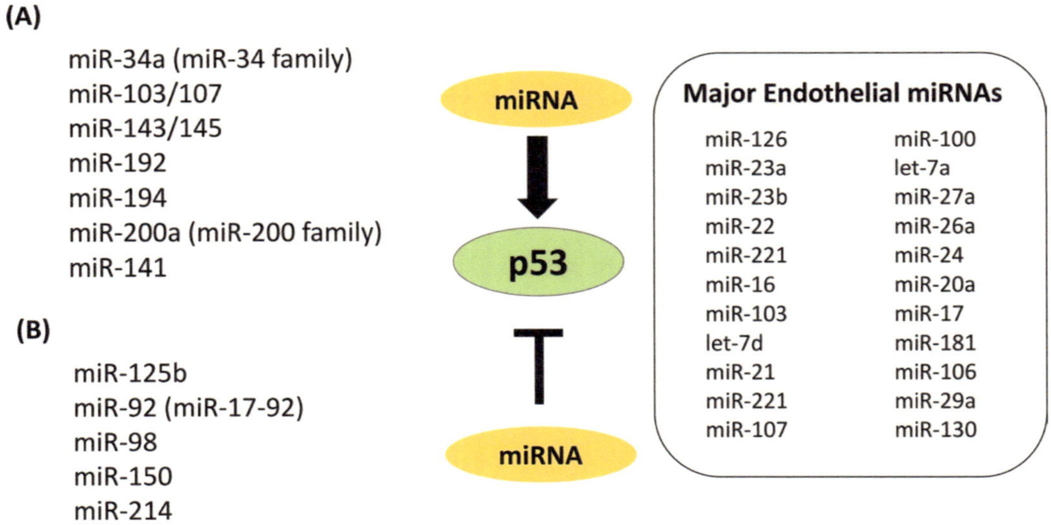

Figure 5. Endothelial miRNA and p53. (A) Endothelial miRNAs regulated by p53. (B) Endothelial miRNAs directly target p53.

lated by p53 are summarized in Section 4.3. Several miRNAs can modulate the process of miRNA biogenesis. The impact of miRNA biogenesis by transcriptional factors has first reported about transforming growth factor beta (TGF-beta) signaling in 2008 [101]. TGF-beta family orchestrates biological processes in vascular development [102]. Davis et al. demonstrated that smads, downstream transcriptional factors of TGF-beta signaling, play a critical role in processing miRNAs by the RNase III-type protein Drosha in nucleus [101]. Similarly, p53 affects the maturation process of miRNAs. The nuclear RNase III Drosha complex contains Drosha, DiGeorge syndrome critical region gene 8 (DGCR8), and the DEAD box RNA helicases, such as p68 and p72 (DDX5 and DDX17, respectively) [103]. P53 interacts with Drosha through p68, facilitating the process of primary miRNAs into precursor miRNAs [104]. Maturation of some precursor miRNAs from primary miRNAs, such as miR-16-1, miR-143, miR-145, and miR-206, is promoted by Doxorubicin stimulated wild type p53 in colon cancer cell lines, HCT-116. Association between a set of miRNAs and Ago2 protein was controlled by p53 [105]. Activated p53 interacts with AGO2 to affect incorporation of let-7 family members. Moreover, p53 induced RNA-binding-motif protein 38 (RBM38) that determined target mRNA selection with miRNAs [106]. Interestingly, Rbm38 deficient mice were likely to accelerate senescence and prone to spontaneous tumors [107]. All these studies had no data using endothelial cells; however, basic insights would be connected to the future study about p53 and miRNAs in the cardiovascular research.

3.5. Regulation of p53 by miRNAs

Many miRNAs regulate p53 directly and indirectly. Endothelial miRNAs can target p53. More than 20 miRNAs that modulated p53 are reported. Among them, miR-92, miR-25, miR-214, and miR-638 play important roles in endothelial cell (**Figure 5B**).

3.5.1. miR-125b

TGF-beta2 induces endothelial-to-mesenchymal transition (EndMT) [108]. The expression of miR-125b in EndMT-derived fibroblast-like cells is significantly higher compared to that in the original mice endothelial cells [109]. In this experiment, miR-125b elevation was negatively associated with p53 expression after EndMT change. Since p53 is a direct target of miR-125b in several human cells, such as neuroblastoma cells and lung fibroblast cells, downregulated p53 by miR-125b possibly modulate TGF-beta-induced profibrotic signaling in endothelial cells [110]. The expression of miR-125b was altered by cell-matrix adhesion in human mesenchymal stem cells (hMSCs) [111]. miR-125b targeted p53, which regulate survival of hMSCs and endogenous miR-125b increased during reprogramming of mouse embryo fibroblasts (MEFs) to induced pluripotent cells. Indeed, miR-125b was not increased by loss of cell adhesion in HUVEC. Sepsis damages endothelial cells, causing multiple organ failure [81]. Transfection of endothelial cells with miR-125b mimics attenuate LPS-induced ICAM-1 and VCAM-1 expression by inhibiting TRAF6 and NF-κB activation [112]. Induction of miR-125 in mice heart attenuated cecal ligation (CLP)-induced sepsis as well and improved survival. These studies suggest that miR-125b regulates angiogenesis and vascular inflammation.

3.5.2. miR-17-92 cluster

Seven individual mature miRNAs (miR-17-5p, miR-17-3p, miR-18a, miR-19a, miR-19b, miR-20a, and miR-92a) are produced from primary miR-17-92, located in the open reading frame 25 (C13orf25) on chromosome 13 in human (**Figure 4D**). Mice knockout or overexpressing of miR-17-92 cluster died shortly after birth, suggested that the balance of miR-17-92 expression are involved in normal development [113, 114]. Originally, miR-17-92 has shown to be a highly conserved cluster, called oncomir-1, and extensively studied the molecular mechanism of tumorgenesis [115]. The roles of miR-17-92 for cardiovascular diseases have been investigated.

One miRNA of this cluster, miR-92a, blocked angiogenetic function in endothelial cells and inhibition of miR-92a by systemic administration of an antagomir-enhanced neovascularization and functional recovery from damaged tissue in hindlimb ischemic mice model [116]. Inhibition of miR-92a-enhanced endothelial cell proliferation and migration, probably through an increased phosphorylation of ERK1/2, JNK, and eNOS. miR-92a promotes pro-atherogenic changes in endothelial cells [117]. Disturbed flow increased miR-92a level in endothelial cells and miR-92a suppressed KLF2 and phosphatidic acid phosphatase type 2B (PPAP2B) that is involved in coronary artery disease (CAD) by genome-wide association studies (GWAS), driving inflammatory and adhesive endothelial phenotype [117]. Although no reports about miR-17-92 regulation of endothelial p53, according to accumulating data above, miR-17-92 may be involved in vascular events and p53 took some parts in them.

3.5.3. Others: miR-98, miR-150, and miR-214 and beyond

There are many miRNAs that directly regulate p53 in cancer; however, a few in endothelial cells. A variety of miRNAs, including miR-98, miR-150, and miR-214 has been shown to decrease p53 expression in cancer [118]. Hypoxia and reoxygenation conditions promote apoptosis and oxidized low-density lipoprotein (ox-LDL)-induced dysfunction of endothelial cells.

miR-98 rescues these phenomenon by targeting caspase-3 and lectin-like oxidized low-density lipoprotein receptor 1 (LOX-1), respectively [119, 120]. Stromal cell-derived factor 1α (SDF-1α) and its receptor CXCR4 control mobilization and migration of EPC. miR-150 decreased CXCR4 expression, leading to impaired EPC migration [121]. In mice studies, decreased miR-150 in EPC helped to revascularize the ischemic heart. miR-150 affected blood-brain barrier (BBB) permeability. Antagomir-150 treatment protected BBB, reduced infarct volume in post-stroke rat via angiopoietin receptor Tie-2 [122].

Targets of miRNAs are recognized by pairing between the seed sequence of miRNA and complementary sites in target mRNAs. There are many useful tools to search for miRNA target genes. Among them, Targetscan is one of the reliable resources many researchers are widely taking. Targetscan predicts four miRNAs, let-7, miR-22, miR122, and miR-150, which are broadly conserved among vertebrates to bind onto 3′UTR of human p53 mRNA (http://www.targetscan.org/vert_71/). Future studies could reveal the function of these miRNAs and their relationship to p53.

4. Conclusion

miRNAs are crucial regulators of gene expression for diverse physiological and pathological processes. Endothelial miRNAs have been intensively studied since Kuehbacher A et al. released that genetic knockout of Dicer and Drosha, miRNA-processing enzymes, inhibited capillary sprouting of endothelial cells and tube formation [123]. Recently Hratmann P et al. demonstrated that Dicer in endothelial cells promoted atherosclerosis and endothelial inflammation [124]. In contrast, p53 is involved in a variety of diseases, such as vascular remodeling, atherosclerosis, hypertension, and hypoxic pulmonary artery remodeling as well as cancer biology.

The importance of p53 and miRNAs in endothelial cells has been shown here. We demonstrated the regulation of endothelial miRNAs by p53 and the modulation of p53 by miRNAs in endothelial cells. These miRNAs play pivotal roles in vascular development and the onset of cardiovascular diseases. The ubiquitin E3 ligase Mdm2 stimulates p53 degradation, in turn, p53 promotes Mdm2 gene expression. Therefore, there is a negative feedback loop between p53 and Mdm2. miR-192, miR-194, and miR-215 targeted Mdm2 protein, which could disrupt this p53-Mdm2 feedback loop [125]. Future studies will unveil the complex and fascinating pathway and loop composed by p53 and miRNAs and develop therapeutic machinery of vascular diseases.

Author details

Munekazu Yamakuchi[1]*, Sushil Panta[2] and Teruto Hashiguchi[1]

*Address all correspondence to: munekazu@m.kufm.kagoshima-u.ac.jp

1 Department of Laboratory and Vascular Medicine, Graduate School of Medical and Dental Sciences, Kagoshima University, Kagoshima, Japan

2 School of Health and Allied Sciences, Faculty of Health Sciences, Pokhara University, Pokhara-Lekhnath, Nepal

References

[1] Vogelstein B, Kinzler KW. Cancer genes and the pathways they control. Nature Medicine. 2004;**10**(8):789-799. doi: 10.1038/nm1087. PubMed PMID: 15286780

[2] Vousden KH, Prives C. Blinded by the light: The growing complexity of p53. Cell. 2009; **137**(3):413-431. DOI: 10.1016/j.cell.2009.04.037. PubMed PMID: 19410540

[3] Gottlieb TM, Oren M. p53 and apoptosis. Seminars in Cancer Biology. 1998;**8**(5):359-368. PubMed PMID: 10101801

[4] Fields S, Jang SK. Presence of a potent transcription activating sequence in the p53 protein. Science. 1990;**249**(4972):1046-1049. Epub 1990/08/31. PubMed PMID: 2144363

[5] Joerger AC, Fersht AR. The tumor suppressor p53: From structures to drug discovery. Cold Spring Harbor Perspectives in Biology. 2010;**2**(6):a000919. Epub 2010/06/03. DOI: 10.1101/cshperspect.a000919. PubMed PMID: 20516128; PubMed Central PMCID: PMCPMC2869527

[6] Bullock AN, Henckel J, DeDecker BS, Johnson CM, Nikolova PV, Proctor MR, et al. Thermodynamic stability of wild-type and mutant p53 core domain. Proceedings of the National Academy of Sciences of the United States of America. 1997;**94**(26):14338-14342. Epub 1998/02/07. PubMed PMID: 9405613; PubMed Central PMCID: PMCPMC24967

[7] Olivier M, Eeles R, Hollstein M, Khan MA, Harris CC, Hainaut P. The IARC TP53 database: New online mutation analysis and recommendations to users. Human Mutation. 2002; **19**(6):607-614. Epub 2002/05/15. DOI: 10.1002/humu.10081. PubMed PMID: 12007217

[8] Lakin ND, Jackson SP. Regulation of p53 in response to DNA damage. Oncogene. 1999; **18**:7644. DOI: 10.1038/sj.onc.1203015

[9] Komarova EA, Zelnick CR, Chin D, Zeremski M, Gleiberman AS, Bacus SS, et al. Intracellular localization of p53 tumor suppressor protein in gamma-irradiated cells is cell cycle regulated and determined by the nucleus. Cancer Research. 1997;**57**(23):5217-5220. Epub 1997/12/11. PubMed PMID: 9393737

[10] Harris SL, Levine AJ. The p53 pathway: Positive and negative feedback loops. Oncogene. 2005;**24**(17):2899-2908. Epub 2005/04/20. DOI: 10.1038/sj.onc.1208615. PubMed PMID: 15838523

[11] Appella E, Anderson CW. Post-translational modifications and activation of p53 by genotoxic stresses. European Journal of Biochemistry. 2001;**268**(10):2764-2772. Epub 2001/05/19. PubMed PMID: 11358490

[12] Gu W, Roeder RG. Activation of p53 sequence-specific DNA binding by acetylation of the p53 C-terminal Domain. Cell. 1997 Aug 22;**90**(4):595-606. DOI: 10.1016/S0092-8674(00)80521-8

[13] Sheikh MS, Fornace AJ, Jr. Role of p53 family members in apoptosis. Journal of Cellular Physiology. 2000;**182**(2):171-181. DOI: 10.1002/(SICI)1097-4652(200002)182:2<171::AID-JCP5>3.0.CO;2-3. PubMed PMID: 10623880

[14] Jin S, Levine AJ. The p53 functional circuit. Journal of Cell Science. 2001;**114**(Pt 23):4139-4140. Epub 2001/12/12. PubMed PMID: 11739646

[15] Munshi N, Fernandis AZ, Cherla RP, Park IW, Ganju RK. Lipopolysaccharide-induced apoptosis of endothelial cells and its inhibition by vascular endothelial growth factor. Journal of Immunology (Baltimore, MD, 1950). 2002;**168**(11):5860-5866. Epub 2002/05/23. PubMed PMID: 12023390

[16] Donehower LA, Harvey M, Slagle BL, McArthur MJ, Montgomery Jr CA, Butel JS, et al. Mice deficient for p53 are developmentally normal but susceptible to spontaneous tumours. Nature. 1992;**356**(6366):215-221. DOI: 10.1038/356215a0. PubMed PMID: 1552940

[17] Gogiraju R, Xu X, Bochenek ML, Steinbrecher JH, Lehnart SE, Wenzel P, et al. Endothelial p53 deletion improves angiogenesis and prevents cardiac fibrosis and heart failure induced by pressure overload in mice. Journal of the American Heart Association. 2015 Feb 24;**4**(2). pii: e001770. DOI: 10.1161/JAHA.115.001770. PubMed PMID: 25713289; PubMed Central PMCID: PMCPMC4345879

[18] Yokoyama M, Okada S, Nakagomi A, Moriya J, Shimizu I, Nojima A, et al. Inhibition of endothelial p53 improves metabolic abnormalities related to dietary obesity. Cell Reports. 2014;**7**(5):1691-1703. DOI: 10.1016/j.celrep.2014.04.046. PubMed PMID: 24857662

[19] Kumar A, Kim CS, Hoffman TA, Naqvi A, Dericco J, Jung SB, et al. p53 Impairs endothelial function by transcriptionally repressing Kruppel-Like Factor 2. Arteriosclerosis, Thrombosis, and Vascular Biology. 2011;**31**(1):133-141. DOI: 10.1161/ATVBAHA.110.215061. PubMed PMID: 20947822; PubMed Central PMCID: PMCPMC3064482

[20] Panta S, Yamakuchi M, Shimizu T, Takenouchi K, Oyama Y, Koriyama T, et al. Low grade inflammation inhibits VEGF induced HUVECs migration in p53 dependent manner. Biochemical and Biophysical Research Communications. 2017 Feb 5;**483**(2):803-809. DOI: 10.1016/j.bbrc.2016.12.096. PubMed PMID: 27998768

[21] Lukin DJ, Carvajal LA, Liu WJ, Resnick-Silverman L, Manfredi JJ. p53 Promotes cell survival due to the reversibility of its cell-cycle checkpoints. Molecular Cancer Research: MCR. 2015;**13**(1):16-28. Epub 2014/08/28. DOI: 10.1158/1541-7786.mcr-14-0177. PubMed PMID: 25158956; PubMed Central PMCID: PMCPMC4312522

[22] Ross R. Cell biology of atherosclerosis. Annual Review of Physiology. 1995;**57**:791-804. DOI: 10.1146/annurev.ph.57.030195.004043. PubMed PMID: 7778883

[23] Guevara NV, Kim HS, Antonova EI, Chan L. The absence of p53 accelerates atherosclerosis by increasing cell proliferation in vivo. Nature Medicine. 1999;**5**(3):335-339. DOI: 10.1038/6585. PubMed PMID: 10086392

[24] van Vlijmen BJ, Gerritsen G, Franken AL, Boesten LS, Kockx MM, Gijbels MJ, et al. Macrophage p53 deficiency leads to enhanced atherosclerosis in APOE*3-Leiden transgenic mice. Circulation Research. 2001;**88**(8):780-786. PubMed PMID: 11325869

[25] Heinloth A, Brune B, Fischer B, Galle J. Nitric oxide prevents oxidised LDL-induced p53 accumulation, cytochrome c translocation, and apoptosis in macrophages via guanylate cyclase stimulation. Atherosclerosis. 2002;**162**(1):93-101. PubMed PMID: 11947902

[26] Matsushita K, Morrell CN, Cambien B, Yang SX, Yamakuchi M, Bao C, et al. Nitric oxide regulates exocytosis by S-nitrosylation of N-ethylmaleimide-sensitive factor. Cell. 2003;**115**(2):139-150. PubMed PMID: 14567912; PubMed Central PMCID: PMCPMC2846406

[27] Heo KS, Lee H, Nigro P, Thomas T, Le NT, Chang E, et al. PKCzeta mediates disturbed flow-induced endothelial apoptosis via p53 SUMOylation. Journal of Cell Biology. 2011;**193**(5):867-884. DOI: 10.1083/jcb.201010051. PubMed PMID: 21624955; PubMed Central PMCID: PMCPMC3105539

[28] Li JM, Fan LM, George VT, Brooks G. Nox2 regulates endothelial cell cycle arrest and apoptosis via p21cip1 and p53. Free Radical Biology and Medicine. 2007;**43**(6):976-986. DOI: 10.1016/j.freeradbiomed.2007.06.001. PubMed PMID: 17697942; PubMed Central PMCID: PMCPMC2889611

[29] Kim KS, Kang KW, Seu YB, Baek SH, Kim JR. Interferon-gamma induces cellular senescence through p53-dependent DNA damage signaling in human endothelial cells. Mechanisms of Ageing and Development. 2009;**130**(3):179-188. DOI: 10.1016/j.mad.2008.11.004. PubMed PMID: 19071156

[30] Ito T, Yagi S, Yamakuchi M. MicroRNA-34a regulation of endothelial senescence. Biochemical and Biophysical Research Communications. 2010;**398**(4):735-740. DOI: 10.1016/j.bbrc.2010.07.012. PubMed PMID: 20627091

[31] Donato AJ, Magerko KA, Lawson BR, Durrant JR, Lesniewski LA, Seals DR. SIRT-1 and vascular endothelial dysfunction with ageing in mice and humans. Journal of Physiology. 2011;**589**(Pt 18):4545-4554. DOI: 10.1113/jphysiol.2011.211219. PubMed PMID: 21746786; PubMed Central PMCID: PMCPMC3208223

[32] Luo J, Nikolaev AY, Imai S, Chen D, Su F, Shiloh A, et al. Negative control of p53 by Sir2alpha promotes cell survival under stress. Cell. 2001;**107**(2):137-148. PubMed PMID: 11672522

[33] Vaziri H, Dessain SK, Ng Eaton E, Imai SI, Frye RA, Pandita TK, et al. hSIR2(SIRT1) functions as an NAD-dependent p53 deacetylase. Cell. 2001;**107**(2):149-159. PubMed PMID: 11672523

[34] Thoreen CC, Sabatini DM. AMPK and p53 help cells through lean times. Cell Metabolism. 2005;**1**(5):287-288. DOI: 10.1016/j.cmet.2005.04.009. PubMed PMID: 16054073

[35] Feng Z, Zhang H, Levine AJ, Jin S. The coordinate regulation of the p53 and mTOR pathways in cells. Proceedings of the National Academy of Sciences of the United States of America. 2005;**102**(23):8204-8209. DOI: 10.1073/pnas.0502857102. PubMed PMID: 15928081; PubMed Central PMCID: PMCPMC1142118

[36] Mizuno S, Bogaard HJ, Kraskauskas D, Alhussaini A, Gomez-Arroyo J, Voelkel NF, et al. p53 gene deficiency promotes hypoxia-induced pulmonary hypertension and vascular remodeling in mice. American Journal of Physiology. Lung Cellular and Molecular Physiology. 2011;**300**(5):L753-L761. DOI: 10.1152/ajplung.00286.2010. PubMed PMID: 21335523

[37] Yoshida T, Kaestner KH, Owens GK. Conditional deletion of Kruppel-like factor 4 delays downregulation of smooth muscle cell differentiation markers but accelerates neointimal formation following vascular injury. Circulation Research. 2008;**102**(12):1548-1557. DOI: 10.1161/CIRCRESAHA.108.176974. PubMed PMID: 18483411; PubMed Central PMCID: PMCPMC2633447

[38] Porrello ER, Olson EN. A neonatal blueprint for cardiac regeneration. Stem Cell Research. 2014;**13**(3, Part B):556-570. DOI: 10.1016/j.scr.2014.06.003

[39] Chen HW, Yu SL, Chen WJ, Yang PC, Chien CT, Chou HY, et al. Dynamic changes of gene expression profiles during postnatal development of the heart in mice. Heart. 2004;**90**(8):927-934. DOI: 10.1136/hrt.2002.006734. PubMed PMID: PMC1768375

[40] Senyo SE, Steinhauser ML, Pizzimenti CL, Yang VK, Cai L, Wang M, et al. Mammalian heart renewal by preexisting cardiomyocytes. Nature. 2013;**493**(7432):433-436. DOI: 10.1038/nature11682. PubMed PMID: PMC3548046

[41] Bergmann O, Bhardwaj RD, Bernard S, Zdunek S, Barnabé-Heider F, Walsh S, et al. Evidence for cardiomyocyte renewal in humans. Science (New York, NY). 2009;**324**(5923):98-102. DOI: 10.1126/science.1164680. PubMed PMID: PMC2991140

[42] Levkau B, Schafers M, Wohlschlaeger J, von Wnuck Lipinski K, Keul P, Hermann S, et al. Survivin determines cardiac function by controlling total cardiomyocyte number. Circulation 2008;**117**(12):1583-1593. Epub 2008/03/12. DOI: 10.1161/circulationaha.107.734160. PubMed PMID: 18332262

[43] Sheng L, Wan B, Feng P, Sun J, Rigo F, Bennett CF, et al. Downregulation of Survivin contributes to cell-cycle arrest during postnatal cardiac development in a severe spinal muscular atrophy mouse model. Human Molecular Genetics. 2018 Feb 1;**27**(3):486-498. DOI: 10.1093/hmg/ddx418

[44] Mirza A, McGuirk M, Hockenberry TN, Wu Q, Ashar H, Black S, et al. Human survivin is negatively regulated by wild-type p53 and participates in p53-dependent apoptotic pathway. Oncogene. 2002;**21**(17):2613-2622. Epub 2002/04/20. DOI: 10.1038/sj.onc.1205353. PubMed PMID: 11965534

[45] Engel FB, Schebesta M, Duong MT, Lu G, Ren S, Madwed JB, et al. p38 MAP kinase inhibition enables proliferation of adult mammalian cardiomyocytes. Genes & Development. 2005;**19**(10):1175-1187. DOI: 10.1101/gad.1306705. PubMed PMID: PMC1132004

[46] Engel FB, Hsieh PCH, Lee RT, Keating MT. FGF1/p38 MAP kinase inhibitor therapy induces cardiomyocyte mitosis, reduces scarring, and rescues function after myocardial infarction. Proceedings of the National Academy of Sciences of the United States of America. 2006;**103**(42):15546-15551. DOI: 10.1073/pnas.0607382103. PubMed PMID: PMC1622860

[47] Toyoda M, Shirato H, Nakajima K, Kojima M, Takahashi M, Kubota M, et al. Jumonji downregulates cardiac cell proliferation by repressing cyclin D1 expression. Developmental Cell. 2003;**5**(1):85-97. Epub 2003/07/11. PubMed PMID: 12852854

[48] Choi JW, Lee KH, Kim SH, Jin T, Lee BS, Oh J, et al. C-reactive protein induces p53-mediated cell cycle arrest in H9c2 cardiac myocytes. Biochemical and Biophysical Research Communications. 2011;**410**(3):525-530. Epub 2011/06/18. DOI: 10.1016/j.bbrc.2011.06.016. PubMed PMID: 21679689

[49] Axtell MJ, Westholm JO, Lai EC. Vive la difference: biogenesis and evolution of microRNAs in plants and animals. Genome Biology. 2011;**12**(4):221. DOI: 10.1186/gb-2011-12-4-221. PubMed PMID: 21554756; PubMed Central PMCID: PMCPMC3218855

[50] Lee Y, Ahn C, Han J, Choi H, Kim J, Yim J, et al. The nuclear RNase III Drosha initiates microRNA processing. Nature. 2003;**425**(6956):415-419. DOI: 10.1038/nature01957. PubMed PMID: 14508493

[51] Ketting RF, Fischer SE, Bernstein E, Sijen T, Hannon GJ, Plasterk RH. Dicer functions in RNA interference and in synthesis of small RNA involved in developmental timing in C. Elegans. Genes & Development. 2001;**15**(20):2654-2659. DOI: 10.1101/gad.927801. PubMed PMID: 11641272; PubMed Central PMCID: PMCPMC312808

[52] Bernstein E, Caudy AA, Hammond SM, Hannon GJ. Role for a bidentate ribonuclease in the initiation step of RNA interference. Nature. 2001;**409**(6818):363-366. DOI: 10.1038/35053110. PubMed PMID: 11201747

[53] Iwakawa HO, Tomari Y. The functions of MicroRNAs: mRNA decay and translational repression. Trends in Cell Biology. 2015;**25**(11):651-665. DOI: 10.1016/j.tcb.2015.07.011. PubMed PMID: 26437588

[54] Djuranovic S, Nahvi A, Green R. miRNA-mediated gene silencing by translational repression followed by mRNA deadenylation and decay. Science. 2012;**336**(6078):237-240. DOI: 10.1126/science.1215691. PubMed PMID: 22499947; PubMed Central PMCID: PMCPMC3971879

[55] Friedman RC, Farh KK, Burge CB, Bartel DP. Most mammalian mRNAs are conserved targets of microRNAs. Genome Research. 2009;**19**(1):92-105. DOI: 10.1101/gr.082701.108. PubMed PMID: 18955434; PubMed Central PMCID: PMCPMC2612969

[56] Bartel DP. MicroRNAs: Target recognition and regulatory functions. Cell. 2009;**136**(2):215-233. DOI: 10.1016/j.cell.2009.01.002. PubMed PMID: 19167326; PubMed Central PMCID: PMCPMC3794896

[57] Calin GA, Dumitru CD, Shimizu M, Bichi R, Zupo S, Noch E, et al. Frequent deletions and down-regulation of micro- RNA genes miR15 and miR16 at 13q14 in chronic lymphocytic leukemia. Proceedings of the National Academy of Sciences of the United States of America. 2002;**99**(24):15524-15529. DOI: 10.1073/pnas.242606799. PubMed PMID: 12434020; PubMed Central PMCID: PMCPMC137750

[58] Hammond SM. RNAi, microRNAs, and human disease. Cancer Chemotherapy and Pharmacology. 2006;**58**(Suppl 1):s63-s68. DOI: 10.1007/s00280-006-0318-2. PubMed PMID: 17093929

[59] O'Donnell KA, Wentzel EA, Zeller KI, Dang CV, Mendell JT. C-Myc-regulated microRNAs modulate E2F1 expression. Nature. 2005;**435**(7043):839-843. DOI: 10.1038/nature03677. PubMed PMID: 15944709

[60] Chang TC, Wentzel EA, Kent OA, Ramachandran K, Mullendore M, Lee KH, et al. Transactivation of miR-34a by p53 broadly influences gene expression and promotes apoptosis. Molecular Cell. 2007;**26**(5):745-752. DOI: 10.1016/j.molcel.2007.05.010. PubMed PMID: 17540599; PubMed Central PMCID: PMCPMC1939978

[61] Raver-Shapira N, Marciano E, Meiri E, Spector Y, Rosenfeld N, Moskovits N, et al. Transcriptional activation of miR-34a contributes to p53-mediated apoptosis. Molecular Cell. 2007;**26**(5):731-743. DOI: 10.1016/j.molcel.2007.05.017. PubMed PMID: 17540598

[62] Tarasov V, Jung P, Verdoodt B, Lodygin D, Epanchintsev A, Menssen A, et al. Differential regulation of microRNAs by p53 revealed by massively parallel sequencing: miR-34a is a p53 target that induces apoptosis and G1-arrest. Cell Cycle. 2007;**6**(13):1586-1593. DOI: 10.4161/cc.6.13.4436. PubMed PMID: 17554199

[63] He L, He X, Lim LP, de Stanchina E, Xuan Z, Liang Y, et al. A microRNA component of the p53 tumour suppressor network. Nature. 2007;**447**(7148):1130-1134. DOI: 10.1038/nature05939. PubMed PMID: 17554337; PubMed Central PMCID: PMCPMC4590999

[64] Bommer GT, Gerin I, Feng Y, Kaczorowski AJ, Kuick R, Love RE, et al. p53-mediated activation of miRNA34 candidate tumor-suppressor genes. Current Biology. 2007;**17**(15):1298-1307. DOI: 10.1016/j.cub.2007.06.068. PubMed PMID: 17656095

[65] He L, He X, Lowe SW, Hannon GJ. microRNAs join the p53 network--another piece in the tumour-suppression puzzle. Nature Reviews. Cancer. 2007;**7**(11):819-822. DOI: 10.1038/nrc2232. PubMed PMID: 17914404; PubMed Central PMCID: PMCPMC4053212

[66] Maes OC, Sarojini H, Wang E. Stepwise up-regulation of microRNA expression levels from replicating to reversible and irreversible growth arrest states in WI-38 human fibroblasts. Journal of Cellular Physiology. 2009;**221**(1):109-119. DOI: 10.1002/jcp.21834. PubMed PMID: 19475566

[67] Fujita K, Mondal AM, Horikawa I, Nguyen GH, Kumamoto K, Sohn JJ, et al. p53 Isoforms Delta133p53 and p53beta are endogenous regulators of replicative cellular senescence. Nature Cell Biology. 2009;**11**(9):1135-1142. DOI: 10.1038/ncb1928. PubMed PMID: 19701195; PubMed Central PMCID: PMCPMC2802853

[68] Zhao T, Li J, Chen AF. MicroRNA-34a induces endothelial progenitor cell senescence and impedes its angiogenesis via suppressing silent information regulator 1. American Journal of Physiology. Endocrinology and Metabolism. 2010;**299**(1):E110-E116. DOI: 10.1152/ajpendo.00192.2010. PubMed PMID: 20424141; PubMed Central PMCID: PMCPMC2904051

[69] Yamakuchi M, Lowenstein CJ. MiR-34, SIRT1 and p53: The feedback loop. Cell Cycle. 2009;**8**(5):712-715. DOI: 10.4161/cc.8.5.7753. PubMed PMID: 19221490

[70] Gridley T. Notch signaling in vascular development and physiology. Development. 2007;**134**(15):2709-2718. DOI: 10.1242/dev.004184. PubMed PMID: 17611219

[71] Yuan HY, Zhou CB, Chen JM, Liu XB, Wen SS, Xu G, et al. MicroRNA-34a targets regulator of calcineurin 1 to modulate endothelial inflammation after fetal cardiac bypass in goat placenta. Placenta. 2017;**51**:49-56. DOI: 10.1016/j.placenta.2017.01.128. PubMed PMID: 28292468

[72] Fan W, Fang R, Wu X, Liu J, Feng M, Dai G, et al. Shear-sensitive microRNA-34a modulates flow-dependent regulation of endothelial inflammation. Journal of Cell Science. 2015;**128**(1):70-80. DOI: 10.1242/jcs.154252. PubMed PMID: 25395581

[73] Cheng BB, Qu MJ, Wu LL, Shen Y, Yan ZQ, Zhang P, et al. MicroRNA-34a targets Forkhead box j2 to modulate differentiation of endothelial progenitor cells in response to shear stress. Journal of Molecular and Cellular Cardiology. 2014;**74**:4-12. DOI: 10.1016/j.yjmcc.2014.04.016. PubMed PMID: 24792364

[74] Yamakuchi M, Lotterman CD, Bao C, Hruban RH, Karim B, Mendell JT, et al. P53-induced microRNA-107 inhibits HIF-1 and tumor angiogenesis. Proceedings of the National Academy of Sciences of the United States of America. 2010;**107**(14):6334-6339. DOI: 10.1073/pnas.0911082107. PubMed PMID: 20308559; PubMed Central PMCID: PMCPMC2851979

[75] Finnerty JR, Wang WX, Hebert SS, Wilfred BR, Mao G, Nelson PT. The miR-15/107 group of microRNA genes: Evolutionary biology, cellular functions, and roles in human diseases. Journal of Molecular Biology. 2010;**402**(3):491-509. DOI: 10.1016/j.jmb.2010.07.051. PubMed PMID: 20678503; PubMed Central PMCID: PMCPMC2978331

[76] Rottiers V, Naar AM. MicroRNAs in metabolism and metabolic disorders. Nature Reviews. Molecular Cell Biology. 2012;**13**(4):239-250. DOI: 10.1038/nrm3313. PubMed PMID: 22436747; PubMed Central PMCID: PMCPMC4021399

[77] Trajkovski M, Hausser J, Soutschek J, Bhat B, Akin A, Zavolan M, et al. MicroRNAs 103 and 107 regulate insulin sensitivity. Nature. 2011;**474**(7353):649-653. DOI: 10.1038/nature10112. PubMed PMID: 21654750

[78] Chen Z, Lai TC, Jan YH, Lin FM, Wang WC, Xiao H, et al. Hypoxia-responsive miRNAs target argonaute 1 to promote angiogenesis. The Journal of Clinical Investigation. 2013;**123**(3):1057-1067. DOI: 10.1172/JCI65344. PubMed PMID: 23426184; PubMed Central PMCID: PMCPMC3582133

[79] Li Y, Mao L, Gao Y, Baral S, Zhou Y, Hu B. MicroRNA-107 contributes to post-stroke angiogenesis by targeting Dicer-1. Scientific Reports. 2015;**5**:13316. DOI: 10.1038/srep13316. PubMed PMID: 26294080; PubMed Central PMCID: PMCPMC4543985

[80] Jacobs R, Honore PM, Joannes-Boyau O, Boer W, De Regt J, De Waele E, et al. Septic acute kidney injury: The culprit is inflammatory apoptosis rather than ischemic necrosis. Blood Purification. 2011;**32**(4):262-265. DOI: 10.1159/000330244. PubMed PMID: 21860231

[81] Peters K, Unger RE, Brunner J, Kirkpatrick CJ. Molecular basis of endothelial dysfunction in sepsis. Cardiovascular Research. 2003;**60**(1):49-57. PubMed PMID: 14522406

[82] Wang S, Zhang Z, Wang J, Miao H. MiR-107 induces TNF-alpha secretion in endothelial cells causing tubular cell injury in patients with septic acute kidney injury. Biochemical and Biophysical Research Communications. 2017;**483**(1):45-51. DOI: 10.1016/j.bbrc.2017.01.013. PubMed PMID: 28063928

[83] Wang WX, Rajeev BW, Stromberg AJ, Ren N, Tang G, Huang Q, et al. The expression of microRNA miR-107 decreases early in Alzheimer's disease and may accelerate disease progression through regulation of beta-site amyloid precursor protein-cleaving enzyme 1. The Journal of Neuroscience. 2008;**28**(5):1213-1223. DOI: 10.1523/JNEUROSCI.5065-07.2008. PubMed PMID: 18234899; PubMed Central PMCID: PMCPMC2837363

[84] Gheorghiu M, Enciu AM, Popescu BO, Gheorghiu E. Functional and molecular characterization of the effect of amyloid-beta42 on an in vitro epithelial barrier model. Journal of Alzheimer's Disease. 2014;**38**(4):787-798. DOI: 10.3233/JAD-122374. PubMed PMID: 24072066

[85] Wood H. Alzheimer disease: Fibrinogen links amyloid with vascular dysfunction. Nature Reviews. Neurology. 2010;**6**(8):413. DOI: 10.1038/nrneurol.2010.98. PubMed PMID: 20718101

[86] Yao J, Hennessey T, Flynt A, Lai E, Beal MF, Lin MT. MicroRNA-related cofilin abnormality in Alzheimer's disease. PLoS One. 2010;**5**(12):e15546. DOI: 10.1371/journal.pone.0015546. PubMed PMID: 21179570; PubMed Central PMCID: PMCPMC3002958

[87] Kent OA, McCall MN, Cornish TC, Halushka MK. Lessons from miR-143/145: The importance of cell-type localization of miRNAs. Nucleic Acids Research. 2014;**42**(12):7528-7538. DOI: 10.1093/nar/gku461. PubMed PMID: 24875473; PubMed Central PMCID: PMCPMC4081080

[88] Dong P, Xiong Y, Hanley SJB, Yue J, Watari H. Musashi-2, a novel oncoprotein promoting cervical cancer cell growth and invasion, is negatively regulated by p53-induced miR-143 and miR-107 activation. Journal of Experimental & Clinical Cancer Research. 2017;**36**(1):150. DOI: 10.1186/s13046-017-0617-y. PubMed PMID: 29073938; PubMed Central PMCID: PMCPMC5659032

[89] Cordes KR, Sheehy NT, White MP, Berry EC, Morton SU, Muth AN, et al. miR-145 and miR-143 regulate smooth muscle cell fate and plasticity. Nature. 2009;**460**(7256):705-710. DOI: 10.1038/nature08195. PubMed PMID: 19578358; PubMed Central PMCID: PMCPMC2769203

[90] Boettger T, Beetz N, Kostin S, Schneider J, Kruger M, Hein L, et al. Acquisition of the contractile phenotype by murine arterial smooth muscle cells depends on the Mir143/145 gene cluster. The Journal of Clinical Investigation. 2009;**119**(9):2634-2647. DOI: 10.1172/JCI38864. PubMed PMID: 19690389; PubMed Central PMCID: PMCPMC2735940

[91] Elia L, Quintavalle M, Zhang J, Contu R, Cossu L, Latronico MV, et al. The knockout of miR-143 and -145 alters smooth muscle cell maintenance and vascular homeostasis in mice: Correlates with human disease. Cell Death and Differentiation. 2009;**16**(12):1590-1598. DOI: 10.1038/cdd.2009.153. PubMed PMID: 19816508; PubMed Central PMCID: PMCPMC3014107

[92] Lovren F, Pan Y, Quan A, Singh KK, Shukla PC, Gupta N, et al. MicroRNA-145 targeted therapy reduces atherosclerosis. Circulation. 2012;**126**(11 Suppl 1):S81-S90. DOI: 10.1161/CIRCULATIONAHA.111.084186. PubMed PMID: 22965997

[93] Cheng Y, Liu X, Yang J, Lin Y, Xu DZ, Lu Q, et al. MicroRNA-145, a novel smooth muscle cell phenotypic marker and modulator, controls vascular neointimal lesion formation. Circulation Research. 2009;**105**(2):158-166. DOI: 10.1161/CIRCRESAHA.109.197517. PubMed PMID: 19542014; PubMed Central PMCID: PMCPMC2728297

[94] Caruso P, Dempsie Y, Stevens HC, McDonald RA, Long L, Lu R, et al. A role for miR-145 in pulmonary arterial hypertension: Evidence from mouse models and patient samples. Circulation Research. 2012;**111**(3):290-300. DOI: 10.1161/CIRCRESAHA.112.267591. PubMed PMID: 22715469

[95] Deng L, Blanco FJ, Stevens H, Lu R, Caudrillier A, McBride M, et al. MicroRNA-143 activation regulates smooth muscle and endothelial cell crosstalk in pulmonary arterial hypertension. Circulation Research. 2015;**117**(10):870-883. DOI: 10.1161/CIRCRESAHA.115.306806. PubMed PMID: 26311719; PubMed Central PMCID: PMCPMC4620852

[96] Kohlstedt K, Trouvain C, Boettger T, Shi L, Fisslthaler B, Fleming I. AMP-activated protein kinase regulates endothelial cell angiotensin-converting enzyme expression via p53 and the post-transcriptional regulation of microRNA-143/145. Circulation Research. 2013; **112**(8):1150-1158. DOI: 10.1161/CIRCRESAHA.113.301282. PubMed PMID: 23476055

[97] Huang C, Huang J, Ma P, Yu G. microRNA-143 acts as a suppressor of hemangioma growth by targeting Bcl-2. Gene. 2017;**628**:211-217. DOI: 10.1016/j.gene.2017.07.046. PubMed PMID: 28716710

[98] Bai Y, Zhang Y, Hua J, Yang X, Zhang X, Duan M, et al. Silencing microRNA-143 protects the integrity of the blood-brain barrier: Implications for methamphetamine abuse. Scientific Reports. 2016;**6**:35642. DOI: 10.1038/srep35642. PubMed PMID: 27767041; PubMed Central PMCID: PMCPMC5073292

[99] Fuschi P, Carrara M, Voellenkle C, Garcia-Manteiga JM, Righini P, Maimone B, et al. Central role of the p53 pathway in the noncoding-RNA response to oxidative stress. Aging (Albany NY). 2017;**9**(12):2559-2586. DOI: 10.18632/aging.101341. PubMed PMID: 29242407; PubMed Central PMCID: PMCPMC5764393

[100] Magenta A, Cencioni C, Fasanaro P, Zaccagnini G, Greco S, Sarra-Ferraris G, et al. miR-200c is upregulated by oxidative stress and induces endothelial cell apoptosis and senescence via ZEB1 inhibition. Cell Death and Differentiation. 2011;**18**(10):1628-1639. DOI: 10.1038/cdd.2011.42. PubMed PMID: 21527937; PubMed Central PMCID: PMCPMC3172120

[101] Davis BN, Hilyard AC, Lagna G, Hata A. SMAD proteins control DROSHA-mediated microRNA maturation. Nature. 2008;**454**(7200):56-61. DOI: 10.1038/nature07086. PubMed PMID: 18548003; PubMed Central PMCID: PMCPMC2653422

[102] ten Dijke P, Arthur HM. Extracellular control of TGFbeta signalling in vascular development and disease. Nature Reviews. Molecular Cell Biology. 2007;**8**(11):857-869. DOI: 10.1038/nrm2262. PubMed PMID: 17895899

[103] Gregory RI, Yan KP, Amuthan G, Chendrimada T, Doratotaj B, Cooch N, et al. The microprocessor complex mediates the genesis of microRNAs. Nature. 2004;**432**(7014):235-240. DOI: 10.1038/nature03120. PubMed PMID: 15531877

[104] Suzuki HI, Yamagata K, Sugimoto K, Iwamoto T, Kato S, Miyazono K. Modulation of microRNA processing by p53. Nature. 2009;**460**(7254):529-533. DOI: 10.1038/nature08199. PubMed PMID: 19626115

[105] Krell J, Stebbing J, Carissimi C, Dabrowska AF, de Giorgio A, Frampton AE, et al. TP53 regulates miRNA association with AGO2 to remodel the miRNA-mRNA interaction network. Genome Research. 2016;**26**(3):331-341. DOI: 10.1101/gr.191759.115. PubMed PMID: 26701625; PubMed Central PMCID: PMCPMC4772015

[106] Leveille N, Elkon R, Davalos V, Manoharan V, Hollingworth D, Oude Vrielink J, et al. Selective inhibition of microRNA accessibility by RBM38 is required for p53 activity. Nature Communications. 2011;**2**:513. DOI: 10.1038/ncomms1519. PubMed PMID: 22027593; PubMed Central PMCID: PMCPMC3221330

[107] Zhang J, Xu E, Ren C, Yan W, Zhang M, Chen M, et al. Mice deficient in Rbm38, a target of the p53 family, are susceptible to accelerated aging and spontaneous tumors. Proceedings of the National Academy of Sciences of the United States of America. 2014;**111**(52):18637-18642. DOI: 10.1073/pnas.1415607112. PubMed PMID: 25512531; PubMed Central PMCID: PMCPMC4284600

[108] Zeisberg EM, Kalluri R. Origins of cardiac fibroblasts. Circulation Research. 2010; **107**(11):1304-1312. DOI: 10.1161/CIRCRESAHA.110.231910. PubMed PMID: 21106947; PubMed Central PMCID: PMCPMC3098499

[109] Ghosh AK, Nagpal V, Covington JW, Michaels MA, Vaughan DE. Molecular basis of cardiac endothelial-to-mesenchymal transition (EndMT): Differential expression of microRNAs during EndMT. Cellular Signalling. 2012;**24**(5):1031-1036. DOI: 10.1016/j.cellsig.2011.12.024. PubMed PMID: 22245495; PubMed Central PMCID: PMCPMC3298765

[110] Le MT, Teh C, Shyh-Chang N, Xie H, Zhou B, Korzh V, et al. MicroRNA-125b is a novel negative regulator of p53. Genes & Development. 2009;**23**(7):862-876. DOI: 10.1101/gad.1767609. PubMed PMID: 19293287; PubMed Central PMCID: PMCPMC2666337

[111] Yu X, Cohen DM, Chen CS. miR-125b is an adhesion-regulated microRNA that protects mesenchymal stem cells from anoikis. Stem Cells. 2012;**30**(5):956-964. DOI: 10.1002/stem.1064. PubMed PMID: 22331826; PubMed Central PMCID: PMCPMC3323671

[112] Ma H, Wang X, Ha T, Gao M, Liu L, Wang R, et al. MicroRNA-125b prevents cardiac dysfunction in Polymicrobial sepsis by targeting TRAF6-mediated nuclear factor kappaB activation and p53-mediated apoptotic Signaling. The Journal of Infectious Diseases. 2016;**214**(11):1773-1783. DOI: 10.1093/infdis/jiw449. PubMed PMID: 27683819; PubMed Central PMCID: PMCPMC5144735

[113] Ventura A, Young AG, Winslow MM, Lintault L, Meissner A, Erkeland SJ, et al. Targeted deletion reveals essential and overlapping functions of the miR-17 through 92 family

of miRNA clusters. Cell. 2008;**132**(5):875-886. DOI: 10.1016/j.cell.2008.02.019. PubMed PMID: 18329372; PubMed Central PMCID: PMCPMC2323338

[114] Lu Y, Thomson JM, Wong HY, Hammond SM, Hogan BL. Transgenic over-expression of the microRNA miR-17-92 cluster promotes proliferation and inhibits differentiation of lung epithelial progenitor cells. Developmental Biology. 2007;**310**(2):442-453. DOI: 10.1016/j.ydbio.2007.08.007. PubMed PMID: 17765889; PubMed Central PMCID: PMCPMC2052923

[115] Mogilyansky E, Rigoutsos I. The miR-17/92 cluster: A comprehensive update on its genomics, genetics, functions and increasingly important and numerous roles in health and disease. Cell Death and Differentiation. 2013;**20**(12):1603-1614. DOI: 10.1038/cdd.2013.125. PubMed PMID: 24212931; PubMed Central PMCID: PMCPMC3824591

[116] Bonauer A, Carmona G, Iwasaki M, Mione M, Koyanagi M, Fischer A, et al. MicroRNA-92a controls angiogenesis and functional recovery of ischemic tissues in mice. Science 2009;**324**(5935):1710-1713. DOI: 10.1126/science.1174381. PubMed PMID: 19460962

[117] Wu C, Huang RT, Kuo CH, Kumar S, Kim CW, Lin YC, et al. Mechanosensitive PPAP2B regulates endothelial responses to atherorelevant hemodynamic forces. Circulation Research. 2015;**117**(4):e41-e53. DOI: 10.1161/CIRCRESAHA.117.306457. PubMed PMID: 26034042; PubMed Central PMCID: PMCPMC4522239

[118] Deng G, Sui G. Noncoding RNA in oncogenesis: A new era of identifying key players. International Journal of Molecular Sciences. 2013;**14**(9):18319-18449. DOI: 10.3390/ijms140918319. PubMed PMID: 24013378; PubMed Central PMCID: PMCPMC3794782

[119] Li HW, Meng Y, Xie Q, Yi WJ, Lai XL, Bian Q, et al. miR-98 Protects endothelial cells against hypoxia/reoxygenation induced-apoptosis by targeting caspase-3. Biochemical and Biophysical Research Communications. 2015;**467**(3):595-601. DOI: 10.1016/j.bbrc.2015.09.058. PubMed PMID: 26367177

[120] Chen Z, Wang M, He Q, Li Z, Zhao Y, Wang W, et al. MicroRNA-98 rescues proliferation and alleviates ox-LDL-induced apoptosis in HUVECs by targeting LOX-1. Experimental and Therapeutic Medicine. 2017;**13**(5):1702-1710. DOI: 10.3892/etm.2017.4171. PubMed PMID: 28565756; PubMed Central PMCID: PMCPMC5443247

[121] Rolland-Turner M, Goretti E, Bousquenaud M, Leonard F, Nicolas C, Zhang L, et al. Adenosine stimulates the migration of human endothelial progenitor cells. Role of CXCR4 and microRNA-150. PLoS One. 2013;**8**(1):e54135. DOI: 10.1371/journal.pone.0054135. PubMed PMID: 23326587; PubMed Central PMCID: PMCPMC3541240

[122] Fang Z, He QW, Li Q, Chen XL, Baral S, Jin HJ, et al. MicroRNA-150 regulates blood-brain barrier permeability via Tie-2 after permanent middle cerebral artery occlusion in rats. The FASEB Journal. 2016;**30**(6):2097-2107. DOI: 10.1096/fj.201500126. PubMed PMID: 26887441

[123] Kuehbacher A, Urbich C, Zeiher AM, Dimmeler S. Role of dicer and Drosha for endothelial microRNA expression and angiogenesis. Circulation Research. 2007;**101**(1):59-68. DOI: 10.1161/CIRCRESAHA.107.153916. PubMed PMID: 17540974

[124] Hartmann P, Zhou Z, Natarelli L, Wei Y, Nazari-Jahantigh M, Zhu M, et al. Endothelial dicer promotes atherosclerosis and vascular inflammation by miRNA-103-mediated suppression of KLF4. Nature Communications. 2016;**7**:10521. DOI: 10.1038/ncomms10521. PubMed PMID: 26837267; PubMed Central PMCID: PMCPMC4742841

[125] Pichiorri F, Suh SS, Rocci A, De Luca L, Taccioli C, Santhanam R, et al. Downregulation of p53-inducible microRNAs 192, 194, and 215 impairs the p53/MDM2 autoregulatory loop in multiple myeloma development. Cancer Cell. 2010;**18**(4):367-381. DOI: 10.1016/j.ccr.2010.09.005. PubMed PMID: 20951946; PubMed Central PMCID: PMCPMC3561766

Chapter 5

Buerger's Disease: Clinical Aspects and Evidence-Based Treatments

Daniel Guimarães Cacione

Additional information is available at the end of the chapter

http://dx.doi.org/10.5772/intechopen.74603

Abstract

Buerger's disease (thromboangiitis obliterans) is a nonatherosclerotic, segmental, occlusive, and recurring progressive inflammatory form of vasculitis that most commonly affects the small- and medium-sized arteries, veins, and nerves in the upper and lower extremities. The cause is unknown, but it is most common in young men with a history of tobacco abuse. It is responsible for ischemic ulcers and extreme pain in the hands and feet. In many cases, notably in patients with the most severe presentations, there is no possibility of improving the condition with surgery (limb revascularization), and therefore, alternative therapies (e.g., sympathectomy, pharmacological agents, and many others) are used. This chapter discusses clinical aspects of Buerger's disease and evidence-based treatment available currently.

Keywords: thromboangiitis obliterans, vasculitis, limb ischemia, evidence-based treatments

1. Introduction

Thromboangiitis obliterans [Buerger's disease (BD), von Winiwarter disease, thromboangiitis obliterans, presenile gangrene] is a nonatherosclerotic, segmental, occlusive, and inflammatory form of vasculitis that affects arteries with small and medium calibers, veins, and nerves in the upper and lower extremities [1]. Alexander von Winiwarter (Austrian-Belgian surgeon) described one patient with the disease in 1879 [2], but it was Leo Buerger (Austrian-American surgeon), in 1908, who published a complete description of the changes in arteries (intimal thickening, occlusive thrombus, and preservation of arterial architecture) on 11 amputated limbs in young smoker males and named the disease [3].

Buerger's disease (BD) has a global distribution, with a prevalence in patients with peripheral arterial disease (PAD) that ranges from 0.5 (in western Europe) to 66% (Asian countries, such as Japan and Korea) [1, 4, 5].

The etiology remains unknown but involves tobacco exposure (*sine qua non*), hereditary susceptibility, immune response, and coagulation changes [5]. Currently, a possible infectious role is gaining interest, especially after the findings of bacteria of the oral flora in occlusive thrombi in patients with Buerger's disease and moderate to severe periodontitis [6, 7]. Another hypothesis is the possibility of rickettsial infection (associated with environment conditions and genetic susceptibility) in Buerger's disease pathogenesis [8, 9]. Features distinguishing Buerger's disease from atherosclerosis (the main differential diagnosis) include the anatomical distribution of the occlusions (with involvement of both the upper and lower extremities in many cases), associated superficial venous thrombosis, a paucity of atherosclerotic risk factors, and normal proximal large arteries [10].

2. Clinical aspects

The "standard" or the classical profile of Buerger's disease (BD) patient is a young man, aged less than 45–50 years, and a history of previous or current smoking (in about 93% of the patients), presenting symptoms suggestive of ischemia in the distal region of limbs. Usually, ischemia restricted to the lower limb occurs in 74.7% cases, and only in the upper limbs in 20.2% cases, and in both limbs, 5.1% cases [11].

Regarding the degree of ischemia in patients with BD at admission, there is a prevalence of the most advanced degrees, and pain at rest may appear in 23.9% of cases, and ischemic ulcers and gangrene in 38% cases [11]. Intermittent claudication occurs in about 30% of cases, typically as "foot claudication," because of the more distal distribution of the disease.

Other signs and symptoms may occur, such as purpura or flushing of the extremities, coldness, migratory thrombophlebitis (16–38%) [1, 11], Raynaud's phenomenon (44%) [1], and rheumatic manifestations in joints in 12.5% usually preceding the ischemic condition. The Allen test is abnormal in 63% of the cases [1].

The frequency of arterial involvement has been demonstrated in the study by Sasaki et al. [12], including 825 patients from a national survey of intractable vasculitis in Japan. The distribution of arterial disease in this national survey presented a higher prevalence of the disease in the lower extremities presenting in the order of frequency as the anterior tibial (41.4%) and posterior tibial arteries (40.4%), followed by the dorsalis pedis artery (21.2%), fibular (18.4%), and popliteal (18.2%) in the lower extremities. In the upper extremities, there exists predominance of ulnar arteries (11.5%), digital arteries (8.1%), and radial arteries (7.0%). Left or right limb preference was not observed. The involvement of visceral, cerebral, coronary, and internal thoracic arteries is uncommon.

Because of the lack of clinical or laboratory indicators of Buerger's disease and the frequent difficulty in differentiating thromboangiitis obliterans from other vascular pathologies that

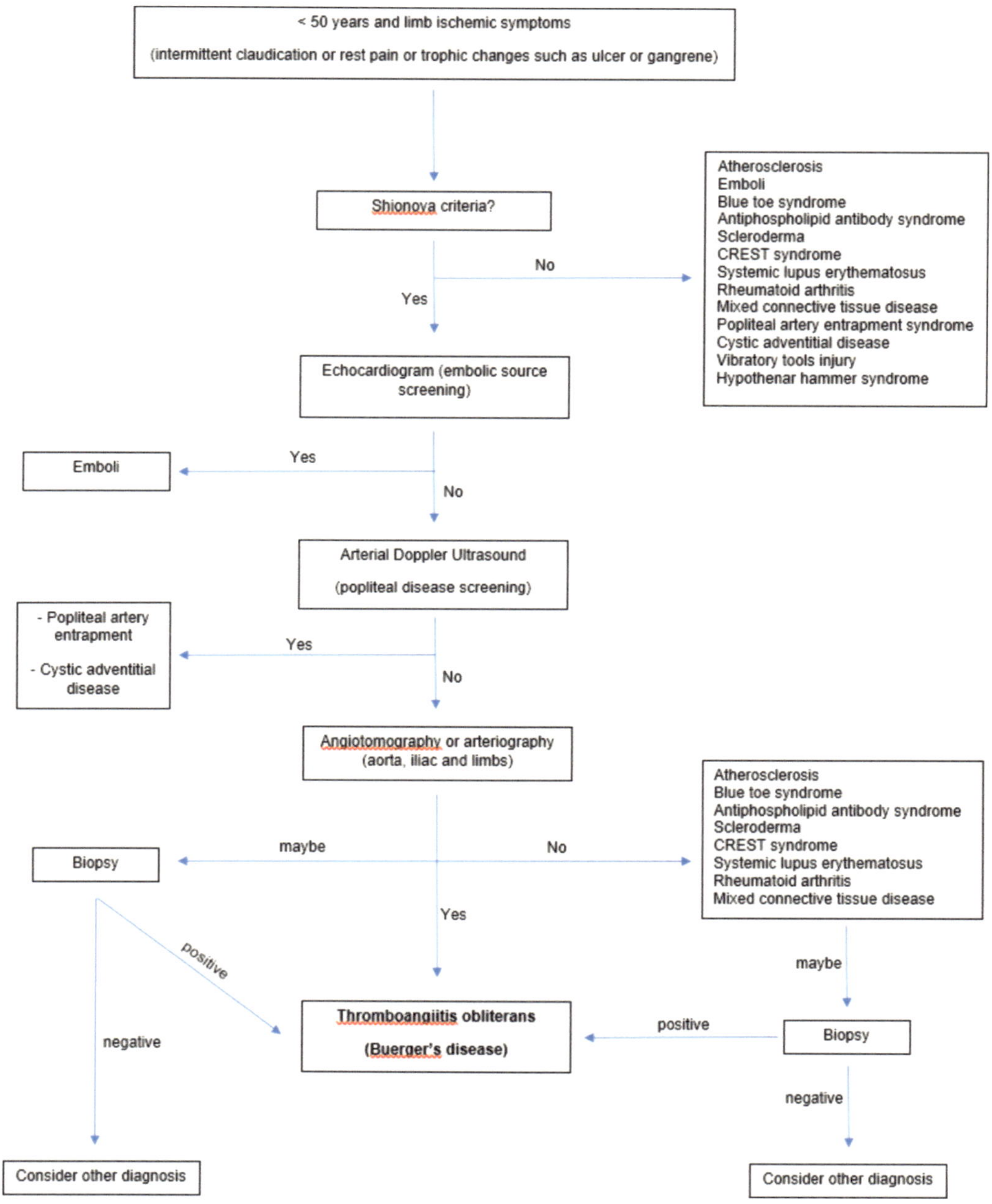

Figure 1. Fluxogram for the diagnosis of Buerger's disease.

might affect the extremities, a number of criteria have been published. The simplest criterion is Shionoya [13], which consists of the presence of five mandatory items: (1) history of smoking, (2) beginning before the age of 50, (3) infrapopliteal occlusive lesions, (4) involvement of upper limbs or migratory phlebitis, and (5) absence of atherosclerotic risk factors, with the exception of smoking. Subsequently, other criteria were elaborated, such as those of Papa and Adar [14], Mills and Porter [15], Olin [1], and the Ministry of Health of Japan [12]. Basically, in addition to the clinical criteria for inclusion by Shionoya, exclusion criteria were added to the findings by noninvasive, angiographic, and histopathological methods (biopsy) to establish the diagnosis.

The use of ultrasound (echocardiogram, arterial, and venous Doppler) is a useful diagnostic tool for the radiographic exclusion of a possible embolic etiology (valvular heart disease, aortic aneurysm, or atherosclerotic) that can mimic the distal ischemia of BD and promote a topography of occlusion and other findings, such as arterial collateralization and phlebitis [1].

Arteriography is an important image examination for confirming the diagnosis of Buerger's disease [16]. Examination findings, which suggest thromboangiitis, include multiple segmental occlusions of the medium- and small-size arteries, mainly below the knee line and elbows, and the presence of collateral arteries adjacent to the areas of occlusion, classically described as a "corkscrew" shape (Martorell's sign) [5, 16].

Biopsy is not routine in the diagnosis of thromboangiitis obliterans, reserved for cases of diagnostic doubt [1]. The histological findings depend on the stage of the disease: in the acute phase, it includes occlusive thrombus with inflammatory characteristics and high cellularity, but with less inflammation in the walls of the blood vessels. Polymorphonuclear leukocytes, micro-abscesses, and multinucleated giant cells may exist in the intermediate phase, in which there is a progressive organization of the thrombus in the arteries and veins. Finally, in established disease, there is a well-organized thrombus with fibrosis [17].

Figure 1 illustrates a suggested fluxogram for the diagnosis of Buerger's disease.

3. Evidence-based treatments

Before studying the types of treatment for Buerger's disease, it is important to present the evidence-based method of evaluation based on the Grading of Recommendations Assessment, Development and Evaluation (GRADE) adopted in this chapter. The GRADE (Grading of Recommendations Assessment, Development and Evaluation) Working Group, formed since the year 2000 by health professionals around the world who research on health evidences, has developed a quality-of-evidence classification system [18]. The quality of a body of evidence defined by GRADE involves consideration of the risk of bias, the objectivity of the results obtained, the heterogeneity of the studies, the precision of the effect estimates, and the risk of publication bias. The GRADE system implies an evaluation of the quality of a body of evidence for each individual outcome and, consequently, how sure the authors are about the efficacy (direction and magnitude) of some intervention [19].

Evidence quality grades are classified as high, moderate, low, and very low. For research on drug efficacy, for example, the highest level of evidence is obtained through randomized controlled clinical trials [19]. From the findings of these trials for a given outcome (e.g., pain at rest), the degree of evidence may vary. Some factors may decrease the strength of evidence, such as studies with a high risk of bias, results obtained through indirect findings (e.g., through comparisons between two interventions that were not confronted in the same study, but in different studies of meta-analysis), presence of heterogeneity in meta-analysis of studies or inconsistencies in the data collected, inaccuracy of results obtained (e.g., a very wide confidence interval), and a high probability of publication bias [19]. Other factors, however, may increase the strength of evidence such as a large magnitude of effect (very high or very low relative risk, well away from the null hypothesis) and gradient-dose response [19]. Thus, after analysis of the potential factors that might strengthen or weaken a given evidence for a specific outcome, the level of evidence available up to that moment is determined [19]. The GRADE Working Group definitions for grading the quality of evidence are among the commonly used definitions illustrating a high, moderate, low, and very low-quality definitions as follows [19]:

"**High** = Further research is very unlikely to change our confidence in the estimate of effect.

Moderate = Further research is likely to have an important impact on our confidence in the estimate of effect and may change the estimate.

Low = Further research is very likely to have an important impact on our confidence in the estimate of effect and is likely to change the estimate.

Very low = Any estimate of effect is very uncertain."

3.1. Overview of the treatments

The treatment of patients with Buerger's disease is based primarily on the complete abolition of smoking. Concomitantly, depending on the degree of ischemia, the measurements are similar to those adopted in patients with peripheral occlusive arterial disease of atherosclerotic etiology: in patients with intermittent claudication, the performance of scheduled exercises, for patients with critical ischemia (rest pain or trophic lesions), provides conditions that increase limb perfusion (revascularization, sympathectomies, pharmacological agents, etc.), as well as analgesia and wound and extremity care.

3.2. Arterial revascularization

The surgical revascularization of limbs in patients with BD is controversial due to the high index of graft occlusion. The important distal involvement of Buerger's disease greatly impairs surgery and long-term patency [5]. Sasajima et al. [20], who present the Japanese experience of 18 years in revascularization in the infra-inguinal territory in patients with thromboangiitis, report the performance of 71 autologous vein grafts in 61 patients with BD and the occurrence of 38 (53%) graft occlusions. Among the possible causes for the high rate of graft failure is the fact that the distal anastomosis is usually performed in diseased artery and subject to frequent vasospasm, the progression of the inflammatory disease itself, the use of veins with "low quality" (because they are also affected by inflammation), and vein stenosis due to myointimal hyperplasia. Among studies about arterial revascularization, figures about a 1-year patency are around 60%. However, because of the design of the studies (prospective and retrospective case series), the evidence is **very low**.

Microsurgical delivery is performed in cases after successful revascularization, in order to reduce the recovery time of patients with superficial gangrene or ischemic ulcers [21]. However, as observed in arterial revascularization, because of the design of the studies (case series), the evidence is **very low**.

3.3. Lumbar sympathectomy

Surgical treatment through lumbar sympathectomy is a surgical modality used to prevent amputations and for alleviation of pain at rest through the vasodilatory effects, resulting from a decreased sympathetic response in the affected limb. Nakajima [22] reports improvement of up to 60% in symptoms in TAO patients according to personal experience. However, the current importance is diminished, due to the unproven effects of amputation prevention and effectiveness in the treatment of pain [22–24].

3.4. Pharmacological treatment

Pharmacological treatment in patients with Buerger's disease is an alternative for selected cases when the disease presents as diffuse and severe limb ischemia. Such critical presentation possibilities for revascularization are markedly diminished; therefore, pharmacological agents are used to improve perfusion.

Selected agents often prescribed for patients such as aspirin, cilostazol, prostanoids, and bosentan are discussed in the subsequent text.

Aspirin [25] is a drug with antiplatelet and anti-inflammatory properties often used to prevent further arterial occlusion. Pharmacologically, aspirin inhibits cyclooxygenase, the enzyme responsible for the synthesis of thromboxane and prostaglandins. Contraindications are hypersensitivity to salicylates, active gastrointestinal ulcers, use in children, patients with active hemorrhage, renal and hepatic failure, and pregnancy. Aspirin is given orally (after meals) at a recommended dosage of 75–325 mg (often 100 mg).

Cilostazol [26, 27] is a pharmacological agent frequently prescribed to patients with peripheral arterial occlusive disease of atherosclerotic etiology [Food and Drug Administration (FDA) approved in 1999). Pharmacologically, cilostazol is the derivative of quinolinone, a drug that inhibits specifically the type III cellular phosphodiesterase, which affects reversible inhibition of platelet aggregation and unequally vasodilatation of the vascular beds (femoral arterial bed is more dilatated than vertebral, carotid, or splanchnic). In other words, cilostazol "steals" a small part of the blood from other territories (gastrointestinal and cerebral) to improve perfusion in ischemic limbs. Cilostazol is contraindicated in patients with congestive heart failure, hemorrheologic disturbances or current bleeding, such as by gastrointestinal or intracranial bleeding, and in individuals with known or suspected hypersensitivity to cilostazol. Side effects of cilostazol include headache, diarrhea, abnormal stools, and tachycardia. Cilostazol is given orally and fasting, at a dose ranging from 50 to 200 mg per day [28, 29].

Prostanoids [30, 31] (prostaglandin analogs and prostacyclin) are derivatives of eicosanoids and are commonly used in the treatment of numerous diseases, including pulmonary hypertension, sexual impotence and glaucoma, and so on. Prostanoids act by binding to specific receptors in the endothelium (causing vasodilation) and platelets inhibiting platelet aggregation, which causes a transient increase in peripheral perfusion. Arterial vasodilation in ischemic areas increases blood perfusion and, consequently, increases the chances of healing of the ulcer and improves pain at rest. By inhibiting platelet aggregation, the occlusion of small- and medium-sized arteries is prevented and, in theory, also stabilizes the disease. Due to their short half-life, about 2–3 min, these synthetic drugs should be administered by continuous intravenous infusion. The newer stable prostacyclin analogs (e.g., iloprost) with a longer half-life have allowed the oral use of these drugs. The most important contraindications are heart failure (any etiology), intracranial hemorrhage, gastrointestinal disorders, and trauma. Side effects include headache, flushing, malaise, gastrointestinal disorders, and hypotension. The maximum dose of iloprost administered is about 2 ng/kg/min of continuous infusion [31].

Bosentan is a powerful double antagonist of endothelin receptors (types A and B), causing selective vasodilator effects [32]. Bosentan has been used successfully in patients with digital ulcers and systemic sclerosis [33–35]. Some important reported side effects are hepatotoxicity and fluid retention. Bosentan is given orally, primarily in patients with pulmonary arterial hypertension, with a recommended dose of 62.5 (twice daily) or 125 mg (twice daily) [32].

It is important to cite the degree of evidence of these treatments. In a recent Cochrane systematic review on the pharmacological treatment of thromboangiitis [36], prostacyclin analog versus placebo, aspirin, and a prostaglandin analog, and folic acid versus placebo were included. Studies that evaluated pharmacological agents such as cilostazol, clopidogrel, and pentoxifylline, or studies that compared oral prostanoid versus intravenous prostanoid were not incorporated because they were not randomized controlled trials. Moderate evidence (one study) suggested that intravenous iloprost was effective in participants with critical limb ischemia (ulcers and rest pain) after 4 weeks of treatment when compared with aspirin, without differences in amputation rates [36]. Two trials indicate that prostacyclin was very effective as prostaglandin analogs in healing ulcers (very low-quality evidence) and extinguishing pain at rest (low-quality evidence), but rates of amputation were not reported by the authors [36]. Moderate evidence (one study) suggested that there was no difference between placebo and the oral prostacyclin analog iloprost (200 and 400 μg) in healing ischemic ulcers or eradicating pain at rest after 8 weeks and 6 months, and rates of amputation after 6 months [36]. Very-low-quality evidence from one study showed no difference between placebo and folic acid, in patients with thromboangiitis obliterans and hyperhomocysteinemia (abnormally high level of homocysteine in the blood), and in rates of amputation and pain scores [36]. Treatment side effects, such as headaches or nausea, were not considered serious [36].

Other pharmacological agents used are those that act on hemorrhagic properties in order to decrease the likelihood of thrombosis, such as dextran and pentoxifylline, arterial vasodilators such as calcium channel blockers and those with anti-inflammatory action in general, such as nonsteroidal anti-inflammatory drugs, phenylbutazone, cyclophosphamide, and corticosteroids. Still other drugs, used in patients with occlusive arterial disease of atherosclerotic etiology, such as carbamate pyridinol and inositol niacinate, have already been used [1]. All these agents have a low efficacy reported in a series of cases and, therefore, with a **very low** level of evidence.

3.5. Pharmacological treatment versus lumbar sympathectomy

The comparison of lumbar sympathectomy, one of the most used treatments in patients with thromboangiitis obliterans with ischemic ulcers and pain at rest with other therapies, was carried out by a recently published systematic review [37] with a finding of "**Very low** evidence suggests that intravenous iloprost (prostacyclin analogue) is more effective than the lumbar sympathectomy in the healing of ischemic ulcers and pain at rest in patients with Buerger's disease. Therefore, until now, the preference of the use of iloprost over the lumbar sympathectomy (and vice versa) is not supported by strong evidence for its routine use. In other words, disponibility and cost may interfere in clinical decision, without evidence supporting both therapies."

3.6. Other treatments

Omental transference, also known as omental transplantation and omentopexy, is a modality of revascularization whose greater omentum is elongated, preserving the native vascularization and then located distally to the ischemic member through a subcutaneous tunnel connecting the abdomen and the foot. The mechanism whose omentum promotes angiogenesis is unknown. Indian and Russian groups of researchers published good results with the technique, with highlights to the works of Singh [38] (reaching 88% of ulcer healing) and Talwar [39] (100% of limb salvage in 62 patients). However, because of the design of the studies (prospective case series), the evidence is **very low**.

Venous arterialization may be defined as the use of the disease-free venous bed as an alternative conduit for perfusion of the peripheral tissues with arterial blood. Meta-analysis of 56 studies (228 patients) published in 2006 [40] about venous arterialization demonstrated that the overall 1-year foot preservation was 71% and the secondary patency of 46% with the use of the technique. However, problems with studies (only six studies were observational and only one was controlled), mixed etiologies of limb ischemia (thromboangiitis and atherosclerosis were evaluated together) and the low number of patients, classified the evidence as **very low**.

The use of stem cells, especially bone marrow derivatives [41], umbilical cord [42], or even adipose tissue, has been the subject of many studies lately. Basically, the progenitor cells are collected, separated, and purified to be injected into the ischemic limb. This has been reported to improve pain at rest, increased healing of ulcers (about 83%) in the study by Durdu et al. [43] and the quality of life of patients undergoing this therapy.

The mobilization and in situ implantation of bone marrow cells, without the need for their processing, can also be performed through bone fenestration (tibia bone), a procedure first described as "revascularization by osteotrepanation" and that stimulates the formation of collateral circulation in the ischemic limb [44]. Allied to this technique, it can stimulate the production of endothelial progenitors through the subcutaneous injection of colony-stimulating factors [45]. Regarding the evidence of this therapy, there is a systematic review protocol [46] about the subject that was recently published, and soon we will study about the efficacy and degree of evidence of this type of treatment in patients with thromboangiitis obliterans.

Stimulation of the spinal cord for the purpose of improving limb pain and perfusion has been related to the study, without severe complications of the method [47]. However, because of the design of the studies (only case series), the evidence is **very low**.

3.7. Amputation

The final stage for the severely affected limb with Buerger's disease is amputation. A study by Cooper et al. [48] retrospectively assessed the amputation rate in 50 patients with BD listed in the Mayo Clinic patient database from January 1976 to December 1999. The authors concluded that the risk of amputation increases progressively in patients who continue to smoke, with the first amputation occurring on average 15.6 years after diagnosis. The estimated risk is 25% at 5 years, 38% at 10 years, and 46% at 20 years, and the risk of amputation higher is 11% at 5 years, 21% at 10 years, and 23% at 20 years. This study also suggests that the risk of amputation is eliminated after 8 years of cessation of smoking. In a study by Sasaki et al. [11] in a retrospective population study of 850 patients in 1993, they reported that about 25.2% of BD patients had some degree of amputation (greater or less). It also reports a 2.73-fold increase in the risk of amputation among patients who remained smokers.

4. Summary (conclusion)

Buerger's disease (thromboangiitis obliterans) is a debilitating vasculitis to the patient and challenging to the physician, as much to the diagnosis as to the treatment. Evidence for the efficacy of numerous therapeutic modalities until now is scarce, with a trend toward greater efficacy of prostacyclin analogs in the treatment of more advanced levels of ischemia (ulcer and pain at rest). Unanimity, however, refers only to the role of smoking in this vasculitis, both at the beginning of the disease and its perpetuation, making it essential to stimulate smoking cessation to minimize the damage of the disease.

Author details

Daniel Guimarães Cacione

Address all correspondence to: dancac@gmail.com

Division of Vascular and Endovascular Surgery, Department of Surgery, UNIFESP—Escola Paulista de Medicina, São Paulo, SP, Brazil

References

[1] Olin JW. Thromboangiitis obliterans (Buerger's disease). The New England Journal of Medicine. 2000;**343**:864-869

[2] von Winiwarter FA. Peculiar form of endarteritis and endophlebitis with gangrene of the foot [Ueber eine eigenthümliche form von Endarteriitis und Endophlebitis mit Gangrän des fusses]. Archiv für Klinische Chirurgie. 1879;**23**:202-226

[3] Buerger L. Thrombo-angiitis obliterans: A study of the vascular lesions leading to presenile spontaneous gangrene. American Journal of Medicine. 1908;**136**:567-580

[4] Cachovan M. Epidemiology and geographic distribution of the thromboangiitis obliterans [Epidemiologic und geographisches Verteilungsmuster der thromboangiitis obliterans]. In: Stuttgart HH, editor. Thromboangiitis Obliterans Morbus Winiwarter-Buerger. 1988. pp. 31-36

[5] Malecki R, Zdrojowy K, Adamiec R. Thromboangiitis obliterans in the 21st century–A new face of disease. Atherosclerosis. 2009;**206**(2):328-334

[6] Iwai T, Inoue Y, Umeda M, Huang Y, Kurihara N, Koike M, et al. Oral bacteria in the occluded arteries of patients with Buerger disease. Journal of Vascular Surgery. 2005; **42**(1):107-115

[7] Li X, Iwai T, Nakamura H, Inoue Y, Chen Y, Umeda M, et al. An ultrastructural study of *Porphyromonas gingivalis*-induced platelet aggregation 2008. Thrombosis Research. 2008;**122**(6):810-819

[8] Bartolo M, Antignani PL, Todini AR, Ricci G. Buerger's disease: Etiologic role of the rickettsiae? Journal des Maladies Vasculaires. 1987;**12**(1):82-84

[9] Fazeli B. Is rickettsia the key to solving the puzzle of Buerger's disease? Vascular. 2013; **22**(5):393-394

[10] Weinberg I, Jaff MR. Nonatherosclerotic arterial disorders of the lower extremities. Circulation. 2012;**126**(2):213-222

[11] Sasaki S, Sakuma M, Yasuda K. Current status of thromboangiitis obliterans (Buerger's disease) in Japan. International Journal of Cardiology. 2000 Aug 31;**75**(Suppl1):S: 175-181

[12] Sasaki S, Sakuma M, Kunihara T, Yasuda K. Distribution of arterial involvement in thromboangiitis obliterans (Buerger's disease): Results of a study conducted by the intractable vasculitis syndromes research group in Japan. Surgery Today. 2000;**30**(7):600-605

[13] Shionoya S. Diagnostic criteria of Buerger's disease. International Journal of Cardiology. 1998;**66**(Suppl):243-245

[14] Papa MZ, Rabi I, Adar RA. Point scoring system for the clinical diagnosis of Buerger's disease. European Journal of Vascular and Endovascular Surgery. 1996;**11**(3):335-339

[15] Mills JL Sr. Buerger's disease in the 21st century: Diagnosis, clinical features, and therapy. Seminars in Vascular Surgery. 2003 Sep;**16**(3):179-189

[16] Suzuki S, Mine H, Umehara I, Yoshida T, Okada Y. Buerger's disease (thromboangiitis obliterans): An analysis of the arteriograms of 119 cases. Clinical Radiology. 1982; **33**:235-240

[17] Kobayashi M, Sugimoto M, Komori K. Endarteritis obliterans in the pathogenesis of Buerger's disease from the pathological and immunohistochemical points of view. Circulation Journal. 2014;**78**:2819-2826

[18] GRADE Working Group. Grading quality of evidence and strength of recommendations. BMJ: British Medical Journal. 2004;**328**(7454):1490

[19] Higgins JPT, Green S (editors). Cochrane Handbook for Systematic Reviews of Interventions Version 5.1.0. Cochrane Handbook for Systematic Reviews of Interventions [Internet]. 2011 [Updated: March 2011]. Available from: http://handbook-5-1.cochrane.org/ [Accessed: 2017]

[20] Sasajima T, Kubo Y, Inaba M, Goh K, Azuma N. Role of infrainguinal bypass in Buerger's disease: An eighteen-year experience. European Journal of Vascular and Endovascular Surgery. 1997 Feb;**13**(2):186-192

[21] Ikeda K, Yotsuyanagi T, Arai K, Suda T, Saito T, Ezoe K. Combined revascularization and free-tissue transfer for limb salvage in a Buerger disease patient. Annals of Vascular Surgery [Internet]. 2012 Apr [cited 2017 Oct 17];**26**(3):422.e5-422.e8

[22] Nakajima N. The change in concept and surgical treatment on Buerger's disease—Personal experience and review. International Journal of Cardiology. 1998;**66**:S273-S280

[23] Paraskevas KI, Liapis CD, Briana DD, Mikhailidis DP. Thromboangiitis obliterans (Buerger's disease): Searching for a therapeutic strategy. Angiology 2007;**58**:75

[24] Roncon-Albuquerque R, Serrao P, Vale-Pereira R, et al. Plasma catecholamines in Buerger's disease: Effects of cigarette smoking and surgical sympathectomy. European Journal of Vascular and Endovascular Surgery. 2002;**24**:338-343

[25] Brunton LL, Chabner BA, Knollmann BC, editors. Goodman and Gilman's the Pharmacological Basis of Therapeutics. 12th ed. New York: McGraw-Hill Companies; 2011. pp. 977-982

[26] Liu Y, Shakur Y, Yoshitake M, Kambayashi JJ. Cilostazol (pletal): A dual inhibitor of cyclic nucleotide phosphodiesterase type 3 and adenosine uptake. Cardiovascular Drug Reviews. 2001 Winter;**19**(4):369-386

[27] Bedenis R, Stewart M, Cleanthis M, Robless P, Mikhailidis DP, Stansby G. Cilostazol for intermittent claudication. Cochrane Database of Systematic Reviews. 2014 Oct 31;(10):1-50.CD003748. DOI: 10.1002/14651858.CD003748.pub4

[28] US Food and Drug Administration. FDA Approved Drug Products [Internet]. Available from: http://www.accessdata.fda.gov/scripts/cder/drugsatfda/index.cfm?fuseaction=Search.DrugDetails [Accessed: November 25, 2015]

[29] Dindyal S, Kyriakides C. A review of cilostazol, a phosphodiesterase inhibitor, and its role in preventing both coronary and peripheral arterial restenosis following endovascular therapy. Recent Patents on Cardiovascular Drug Discovery. 2009;**4**(1):6-14

[30] Ruffolo AJ, Romano M, Ciapponi A. Prostanoids for critical limb ischaemia. Cochrane Database of Systematic Reviews. 2010 Jan 20;(1):1-60. DOI: 10.1002/14651858.CD006544.pub2

[31] Grant SM, Goa KL. Iloprost. A review of its pharmacodynamic and pharmacokinetic properties, and therapeutic potential in peripheral vascular disease, myocardial ischaemia and extracorporeal circulation procedures. Drugs. 1992;**43**(6):889-924

[32] Weber C, Schmitt R, Birnboeck H, Hopfgartner G, van Marle SP, Peeters PAM, et al. Pharmacokinetics and pharmacodynamics of the endothelin-receptor antagonist bosentanin healthy human subjects. Clinical Pharmacology and Therapeutics. 1996;**60**:124-137

[33] De Haro J, Acin F, Bleda S, Varela C, Esparza L. Treatment of thromboangiitis obliterans (Buerger's disease) with bosentan. BMC Cardiovascular Disorders. 2012;**12**:5. DOI: 10.1186/1471-2261-12-5

[34] Launay D, Diot E, Pasquier E, Mouthon L, Boullanger N, Fain O, et al. Bosentan for treatment of active digital ulcers in patients with systemic sclerosis. La Presse Médicale. 2006;**35**(4 Pt 1):587-592

[35] Matucci-Cerinic M, Denton CP, Furst DE, Mayes MD, Hsu VM, Carpentier P, et al. Bosentan treatment of digital ulcers related to systemic sclerosis: Results from the RAPIDS-2 randomised, double-blind, placebo-controlled trial. Annals of the Rheumatic Diseases. 2011;**70**(1):32-38

[36] Cacione DG, Macedo CR, Baptista-Silva JC. Pharmacological treatment for Buerger's disease. Cochrane Database of Systematic Reviews. 2016 Mar 11;(3):1-39. CD011033. DOI: 10.1002/14651858.CD011033.pub3

[37] Cacione DG, Moreno DH, Nakano LC, Baptista-Silva JC. Surgical sympathectomy for Buerger's disease. JRSM Open [Internet]. 2017;**8**(8):1-8. DOI: http://journals.sagepub.com/ doi/10.1177/2054270417717666

[38] Singh I, Ramteke VK. The role of omental transfer in Buerger's disease: New Delhi's experience. The Australian and New Zealand Journal of Surgery [Internet]. 1996 Jun;**66**(6): 372-376. [Cited 2017 Oct 17]. DOI: http://www.ncbi.nlm.nih.gov/pubmed/8678856

[39] Talwar S, Jain S, Porwal R, Laddha BL, Prasad P. Free versus pedicled omental grafts for limb salvage in Buerger's disease. The Australian and New Zealand Journal of Surgery [Internet]. 1998 Jan [cited 2017 Oct 17];**68**(1):38-40

[40] Lu XW, Idu MM, Ubbink DT, Legemate DA. Meta-analysis of the clinical effectiveness of venous arterialization for salvage of critically ischaemic limbs. European Journal of Vascular and Endovascular Surgery. 2006 May [cited 2017 Oct 17];**31**(5):493-499

[41] Boda Z, Udvardy M, Rázsó K, Farkas K, Tóth J, Jámbor L, Oláh Z, Ilonczai P, Szarvas M, Kappelmayer J, Veréb Z, Rajnavölgyi E. Stem cell therapy: A promising and prospective approach in the treatment of patients with severe Buerger's disease. Clinical and Applied Thrombosis/Hemostasis. 2009 Oct;**15**(5):552-560

[42] Kim SW, Han H, Chae GT, Lee SH, Bo S, Yoon JH, Lee YS, Lee KS, Park HK, Kang KS. Successful stem cell therapy using umbilical cord blood-derived multipotent stem cells for Buerger's disease and ischemic limb disease animal model. Stem Cells. 2006; **24**(6):1620-1626

[43] Durdu S, Akar AR, Arat M, Sancak T, Eren NT, Ozyurda U. Autologous bone-marrow mononuclear cell implantation for patients with Rutherford grade II-III thromboangiitis obliterans. Journal of Vascular Surgery. 2006 Oct [cited 2017 Oct 17];**44**(4):732-739

[44] Zusmanovich FN. A new method for activating the collateral circulation–Revascularization osteotrepanation. Vestnik Khirurgii Imeni I. I. Grekova [Internet]. 1991 May [cited 2017 Oct 17];**146**(5):114-115

[45] Kim D-I, Kim M-J, Joh J-H, Shin S-W, Do Y-S, Moon J-Y, et al. Angiogenesis facilitated by autologous whole bone marrow stem cell transplantation for Buerger's disease. Stem Cells. 2006 May [cited 2017 Oct 17;**24**(5):1194-1200

[46] Cacione DG, Moreno DH. Stem cell therapy for treatment of thromboangiitis obliterans (Buerger's disease). Cochrane Database of Systematic Reviews. 2017;(9):1-11. DOI: 10.1002/14651858.CD012794

[47] Donas KP, Schulte S, Ktenidis K, Horsch S. The role of epidural spinal cord stimulation in the treatment of Buerger's disease. Journal of Vascular Surgery. 2005 May;**41**(5):830-836

[48] Cooper LT, Tse TS, Mikhail MA, McBane RD, Stanson AW, Ballman KV. Long-term survival and amputation risk in thromboangiitis obliterans (Buerger's disease). Journal of the American College of Cardiology. 2004 Dec 21;**44**(12):2410-2411